WATCHING OUR WEIGHTS

WATCHING OUR WEIGHTS

The Contradictions of Televising
Fatness in the "Obesity Epidemic"

MELISSA ZIMDARS

RUTGERS UNIVERSITY PRESS

New Brunswick, Camden, and Newark, New Jersey, and London

Library of Congress Cataloging-in-Publication Data

Names: Zimdars, Melissa, 1985– author.
Title: Watching our weights : the contradictions of televising fatness in the "obesity epidemic" / Melissa Zimdars.
Description: New Brunswick, NJ : Rutgers University Press, [2018] | Includes bibliographical references and index.
Identifiers: LCCN 2018004266 | ISBN 9780813593555 (cloth : alk. paper) | ISBN 9780813593548 (pbk. : alk. paper)
Subjects: LCSH: Obesity on television. | Television—Social aspects—United States. | Obesity—Social aspects.
Classification: LCC PN1992.8.O24 Z56 2018 | DDC 791.45/6561—dc23
LC record available at https://lccn.loc.gov/2018004266

A British Cataloging-in-Publication record for this book is available from the British Library.

♾ The paper used in this publication meets the requirements of the American National Standard for Information Sciences—Permanence of Paper for Printed Library Materials, ANSI Z39.48–1992.

www.rutgersuniversitypress.org

Manufactured in the United States of America

For my parents, Tom and Karla.

Contents

WATCHING OUR WEIGHTS

1   *Televising Fatness*

"On behalf of our chubby trio, I welcome you into our flabby foursome," Ethel says to Lucy, who dramatically responds, "I'm going to go out and kill myself." Lucy, who had gained weight since marrying Ricky, realizes her weight increase only when Ricky, Ethel, and Fred make her step on a scale after she calls Ricky "porky" and "fatso" for eating sixteen oysters. While Ricky, Ethel, and Fred all admit with minimal lament to getting a little "puffy" over the years, Lucy takes the news hard, referring to herself as just a "bunch of blubber." The remainder of "The Diet" (1951) episode of *I Love Lucy* (1951–1957) depicts Lucy running circles around her apartment to lose twelve pounds in four days in order to fit into a dance costume for Ricky's show. In classic *I Love Lucy* form, she also goes on a strict diet of celery that starves her to the point of stealing table scraps from the hopeful dog waiting under the dinner table. Desperate to meet her weight-loss goal, Lucy even sits in a "human pressure cooker" to sweat out the pounds. By episode's end, she achieves her weight-loss goal, but is so delirious and malnourished that a medical doctor orders her to spend three weeks recovering in bed.

On its surface, this episode perpetuates fat and body shaming in relation to characters whom audiences may not even read as fat. In fact, Lucy's goal in the episode is to fit into a size twelve costume, which would be considered a size six or eight by today's fashion standards. "The Diet" also reinforces the notion that fatness is undesirable, that becoming fat is something to be avoided at all costs, even if dieting makes you miserable. Yet, at the same time, the show positions Lucy's weight-reduction techniques as excessive, silly, and even unnecessary. Ricky refers to her as "plump" in a loving rather than denigrating way. And Lucy was not bothered by her body size before stepping on the scale and attaching a number to it, before deciding to fit her body into a costume instead of fitting a costume to her body. Until Lucy allowed external bodily cues from people and clothing to start dictating her worth, she seemed perfectly fine with herself.

This same narrative plays out again and again on television. One episode of *The Odd Couple* (1970–1975), "Fat Farm" (1971), shows Bob convincing Oscar to accompany him to a "fat farm" after watching him eat six hotdogs at a baseball game, "but only chewing two." After his doctor also recommends losing weight to improve his health, Oscar begrudgingly agrees, but jokes, "It embarrasses me to be around all of those fat people because I'm one of them. Nobody wants to see fat birds of a feather flocking together." The nutrition and exercise practices at the "fat farm" prove to be as outrageous as Lucy's attempts to lose weight—they're only allowed to "nibble" on celery and carrots, they're only allowed to eat *imaginary* baked Alaska for dessert because weight is all "in the mind." These restrictive practices push Oscar to smuggle in salami, bread, and cheese, leading to warnings that he's going to be expelled from the "fat farm" and left to deal with his "bad body" on his own. Similarly, Bob on *The Bob Newhart Show* (1972–1978) also desires to lose weight to improve his health per his doctor's advice. Bob's doctor gives him charts to track calories, pamphlets detailing exercises, and a complicated list of foods to avoid, leaving Bob to ask, "Wouldn't it be easier to just stop eating?" Like Lucy and Oscar, Bob goes on a strict diet, but eventually becomes so hungry he wants to "attack everything edible." But by the end of "Fit, Fat, and Forty One" (1973), Bob does lose ten pounds and his wife, Carol, finds him "much sexier this way."

Again, none of these actors would likely be read as fat, especially today, yet these episodes rather straightforwardly reject fatness and fat individuals "flocking together." Airing almost twenty years after *I Love Lucy*, both *The Odd Couple* and *The Bob Newhart Show* add another layer to discussions of weight and dieting, reflecting the social context of the time. When *I Love Lucy* aired "The Diet," fatness was not yet considered a major medical concern; however, from the 1950s to the 1970s concerns over fatness moved from the margins to the mainstream.[1] By today's standards, about 50 percent of the U.S. population could be categorized as overweight in the 1970s, and both fatness *and* fitness became increasingly under the purview of medical experts.[2] Whereas *I Love Lucy* focused on the aesthetic of the body and on reducing one's body size to fit clothing, *The Odd Couple* and *The Bob Newhart Show* overtly link fatness and health status. This is not to say that the appearance of the body became of less concern; rather health concerns increased in prominence as well as legitimacy. Oscar's physician says to him while holding a ceramic heart in his hand, "Fat is the mortal enemy of this amazing machine!" And Bob's doctor tells him, "Every extra pound of fat takes a year off of life." This TV trope can be found in other series of the time too, such as the "Archie's Weighty Problem" (1976) episode of *All in the Family* (1971–1979) and the "Crash Diet" (1978) episode of *CHiPs* (1977–1983), where fatness is referred to as an "insidious killer."

These episodes center narratives of health, weight, and fatness, and they also contain moments that offer important commentary on dieting and the pressures many of us feel to make our bodies smaller. For example, on *The Bob Newhart Show*, when Bob's secretary, Carol, does not respond supportively to his complaints about his water-only lunch, he charges, "You've probably never been on a diet!" Exasperated, Carol responds, "In five minutes I'll have been on a diet for *seven years*." This quip demonstrates the way bodily expectations and experiences are also deeply gendered, with women typically feeling more pressure to be thin.[3] It also reflects the rise of fitness and dieting cultures during the

1970s—referred to as the "cult of slimness"—with the release of Jane Fonda's popular aerobic videos idealizing slender bodies and fitness gyms opening around the country.[4] Around the same time, SlimFast released its first weight-loss shakes, the use of (now illegal) appetite suppressants like Dexatrim soared, and Weight Watchers advertisements filled the pages of women's magazines. But while dieting culture and these medical and health conceptualizations of fatness gained prominence both on and off television, the era also saw emerging pushback against dieting culture as well as declarations that "fat is a feminist issue."[5] Nonetheless, feminist accounts of fat embodiment or critical interrogations of discourses emphasizing weight loss via water-only diets took a lot longer to make it on the small screen in overt ways.

During the early to mid-2000s, television started representing fat individuals with considerably greater frequency. Instead of self-contained diet episodes on sitcoms or reliance on fatness as a source of humor, television began centering fatness, or more often reductions in fatness. Contemporary representations and narratives about fatness are deeply shaped by constructions of the "obesity epidemic," or understandings of fatness as a global health problem both caused by individuals and needing to be solved by individuals. Series like *The Biggest Loser* (2004–2016), *Celebrity Fit Club* (2005–2010), *Fat Camp* (2006), and *Fat March* (2007) all focus on transforming the body from fat to thin through diet and exercise with formats ranging from group competitions and weekly eliminations to a collective weight-loss march from Boston to Washington, D.C. These shows then spawned numerous others—as is television's way—that similarly frame fatness as a problem in need of management and, later, as a disease in need of medical treatment. These television series, along with growing governmental, public health, and medical attention to fatness, legitimize dichotomous discourses of the body, namely that thin bodies are healthy and beautiful while fat bodies are unhealthy and visually displeasing.[6]

Like many identity categories, such as gender, race, or ethnicity, being fat marks one as "other" and becomes a way of maintaining social hierarchies and power for some groups at the expense of others. Like maleness or whiteness, thinness is the default, privileged category, while fatness is marked as oppositional to social and cultural idealizations of the body. Fatness is considered excessive, undisciplined, and thus unhealthy, whereas thinness embodies the virtues of self-discipline, self-control, and health.[7] The belief that the size of our bodies, and thus the health of our bodies, is directly connected to our individual choices is so normalized that it can be considered a kind of "common sense." Contemporary fat-themed television content is dominated by this "common sense" knowledge about fatness as unhealthy, undesirable, and deeply reflective of us as either self-disciplined or undisciplined individuals. By promoting individual changes and expert interventions to transform fat bodies into thin bodies, television not only reinforces these dominant discourses but also works to "govern at a distance" by disciplining bodies on-screen and encouraging audiences at home to reject fatness and indiscipline in favor of thinness and self-discipline.[8]

Yet many of these representations of fatness since the early to mid-2000s are also contradictory and inconsistent, exposing television's own incapacity to completely fulfill this governing role. In fact, television is an increasingly important forum for not only debating and exposing the contradictions inherent in dominant health discourses of fatness in the context of the "obesity epidemic," but also creating space for alternative as well as more radical and resistant discourses of the body. For example, assumptions that health is a personal choice are complicated by medicalized representations of fatness as a disease on shows like *My 600-lb Life* (2012–), which may reduce fat stigma while encouraging bodily sympathy as much as bodily shame. Other recent programs actively celebrating fatness include *Big Sexy* (2011) and *Curvy Girls* (2011–2013), while others actively resist fat stereotypes, such as *Huge* (2010) and *Drop Dead Diva* (2009–2014), or represent fatness as just another type of body like on *Loosely Exactly Nicole* (2017). These programs either reject the fat-to-thin transformation via strict dieting and excessive exercise or reject the fat-to-thin transformation altogether.

These examples are part of a long and important tradition of television programs engaging with and creating space for social, cultural, and political change despite being a relatively conservative medium throughout the broadcast era. While the no-compromises, full-body revolution may not be televised, or at least not just yet, television is a medium that helps shape our views of fatness. Even though a significant portion of fat television currently reflects the status quo or constructions of the "obesity epidemic," that is beginning to change. There are only so many ways to tell the same weight-loss story season after television season, and even though calls for us to diet and exercise our way to thinness seem louder and more frequent than ever, many of us are searching for new and less oppressive ways to think about fatness, weight loss, and our own bodies. And television, according to Elana Levine, continually finds ways to accommodate and incorporate "some of the emergent challenges to dominant norms and values."[9] While this typically means maintaining dominant logics of the "obesity epidemic," it also, as Levine argues, "opens the door for small, incremental instances of social change." For example, Ron Becker traces the proliferation of gay-themed television during the 1990s. Although these representations could be read as "moving, affirming, frustrating, entertaining, and insulting" by queer viewers while contributing to a reactionary "straight panic" in the 2000s, they also positively changed media industry attitudes toward gay material and undoubtedly created space for the wider variety of queer representations on television today.[10] The increasingly diverse representations of fatness, representations that are becoming less connected to weight-loss desires and thin ideals, are also evidence of this process. However, we're likely only at the beginning—with a long way to go—before radical representations of the body become "safe" enough for television outside of niche cable channels. Nevertheless, television operates as both an important site of and a resource for fat cultural politics, and according to Herman Gray, television's illogicalities, inconsistencies, and the like sharpen "our focus on its hegemonic as well as its counterhegemonic potentials."[11]

Differing representations of fatness on television are articulated to different discourses of the body and are emblematic of different strands of television's history. Representations of fatness in the makeover or transformational tradition are rife with intrinsic resistance, or examples where disciplinary and surveillance logics breakdown, expertise is challenged, and participants either fail (despite being surveilled, disciplined, and guided by experts) or refuse to change. These shows represent the collision between cultural demands of the body and health assumptions about fatness, with the complicated realities of the way our bodies function (not to mention television producers needing to build tension and interest in the stories they tell). Other emerging fat, feminist television programs can be considered overtly resistant to these bodily dichotomies, fat stereotypes, and automatic assumptions linking fatness and health status. These representations articulated to discourses of fat acceptance and body positivity address fat shame, stigma, and discrimination and typically frame fat embodiment as neutral—if not something to embrace or celebrate—as opposed to some*thing* to reject. This project thus looks at resistance inherent within representations and narratives of fatness as a global health issue, the intrinsic and overt resistance found across stories of medicalized fatness, and programs by which television producers actively create space for alternative and less oppressive ways of thinking about the body. In order to understand what is both new and all too familiar about the fat-themed television proliferating on our screens, we need to take a brief tour through television's limited fat past.

Television's Limited History of Body Size Diversity

When fat bodies, or at least non–normatively thin bodies, were sometimes present on TV, they were often positioned as the butt of jokes or as punch lines. In fact, many of the jokes about and comebacks to Ralph on *The Honeymooners* (1955–1956) reference his size. He is repeatedly called the chubby one, the big fat one, a blimp, fatso, and "an impersonation of two pounds of bologna in a one pound bag." Similarly, Graham is regularly referred to as chubby and fatty throughout the "Couple of Swells" (1989) episode of *Just the Ten of Us* (1988–1990), and when he "fails" his diet (or, to me, when his diet fails him), his wife jokes, "Honey, I'll always support you . . . even if the furniture won't." On *Married with Children* (1987–1997), Al Bundy regularly makes fun of his fat mother-in-law and is downright cruel to the fat women he encounters to the point where a group bands together and charges him with "crimes against obesity." The large size of the mother of another television Al is also constantly used for laughs on *Home*

Improvement (1991–1999). I could go on and on with more examples of fat jokes, from the overtly insulting to the casual and insidious, on *The Simpsons* (1989–), *Family Guy* (1999–), *How I Met Your Mother* (2005–2014), *The Big Bang Theory* (2007–), and even *30 Rock* (2006–2013), when Jenna sings about her "muffin top." Fat jokes have been, and by most accounts still are, the low-hanging fruit of television comedy.

The fat-to-thin transformation is another common trope that reinforces fat stereotypes. This transformation is exemplified by Monica on *Friends* (1994–2004), Annie on *Community* (2009–2015), and Schmidt on *New Girl* (2011–2018). Across each of these programs former fatness becomes a character development tool used to give context and history to the neuroses, obsessions, and overachiever tendencies of specific characters. Amy Gullage argues that *Friends* positions "Fat Monica" as outside the norm and as sloppy, loud, obnoxious, pathetic, and gluttonous. Gullage further contends that Monica's fat-to-thin body transformation represents "contemporary fears of fatness as always lurking in the shadows and eager to consume the healthy, good (both physically and mentally), and controlled body."[12] These transformations also reinforce the idea that there is a thin person trapped inside each fat person just waiting to get out.[13]

Despite television's history of fat jokes and of reinforcing stereotypes of fat people as gluttonous, lazy, loud, and sloppy, among other personality traits and behaviors, TV as a medium is also described as "friendlier" to fat, at least in comparison to film, because of regular attempts to use fatness to portray characters as "everyday" people who may be more relatable to audiences.[14] From Frank on *Cannon* (1971–1976) and Cliff on *Cheers* (1982–1993) to characters on numerous TV programs throughout the 1990s and 2000s, including Jim on *According to Jim* (2001–2009), Drew on *The Drew Carey Show* (1995–2004), Bill on *Still Standing* (2002–2006), Doug on *King of Queens* (1998–2007), Carl on *Family Matters* (1989–1998), Randy on *My Name Is Earl* (2005–2009), Sean on *Grounded for Life* (2001–2005), Tony on *The Sopranos* (1999–2007), Jeff on *Curb Your Enthusiasm* (1999–), Turtle on *Entourage* (2004–2011), and Cameron on *Modern Family* (2009–), fat men—or at least nonidealized male body types—are more frequently represented on the small screen than fat women.[15] Fat men are even common across animated series, including Fred of *The Flintstones* (1960–1966), Fat Albert of *Fat Albert and the Cosby Kids* (1972–1985), Homer, Chief Wiggum, and Barney of *The Simpsons* (1989–), and Peter of *Family Guy* (1999–). Through the display of "soft bodies" and use of the "bumbling oaf" stereotype, fat men on sitcoms, especially through the 1990s and early 2000s, also potentially represent a "crisis in masculinity" and weakening of patriarchy,[16] although numerous representations of non-fat masculinity are interpreted the same way. Fat sitcom husbands also put forth a form of masculinity that is juvenile and immature,[17] yet one that ultimately appears to be a successful and enviable way to live considering most of these men are married to idealized thin women and most have steady employment and comfortable

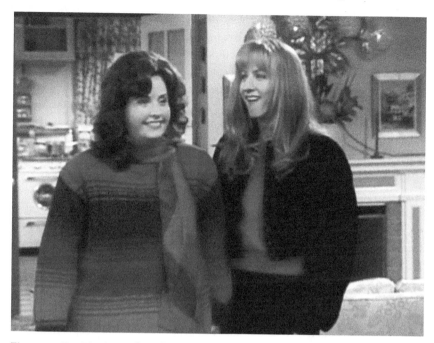

Figure 1   Fat Monica and Rachel on "The One with the Thanksgiving Flashbacks" episode of *Friends* (1998)

homes. The fact that fat women are rarely married to idealized thin men (in this particular heteronormative situation) demonstrates that fat women are typically more bound by hegemonic ideals of beauty.

In fact, TV reflects the gendered ways fatness is experienced and the differing thresholds by which men and women are even considered to be fat, with men perceived as fat when they are seventy pounds "overweight" while women are perceived as fat when they are only ten pounds "overweight."[18] Sandra Bartky argues that fatness, abundance (in height or muscle), or strength in women's bodies is often met with distaste because they defy normative definitions of femininity or womanhood,[19] despite the fact that over half of women can be categorized as "overweight" or "obese."[20] In patriarchal society, women are often denied space, power, and visibility, and fat women inherently transgress those norms as they physically take up more space and are therefore more visible, which implicitly makes fat female bodies appear more powerful and more threatening to patriarchal power hierarchies.[21] Thus, according to Cecilia Hartley, women's bodies are "inscribed as *necessarily thin*," meaning that women must be thin because appearing visibly smaller makes them symbolically weaker.[22] If women do comply with these body norms, or "succeed" in disciplining their bodies by making them visibly smaller and spatially compact, it may gain them interpersonal attention, but rarely respect or social power.[23] These gendered differences of fatness are likely why 33 percent of women-identified characters on television can be categorized as "underweight," at least according to the specious standards set by the body mass index, and why thin women receive more on-screen compliments about their physical appearances compared to fat women. Fat women on TV are also more likely to be insulted compared to thin women.[24] These gendered differences are also why there are far fewer fat women on television overall and why they also tend to be styled less attractively (unkempt hair, bland wardrobe, awkward), desexualized, and positioned as the antithesis to thin characters.[25]

Even though there are more fat men visible throughout television's history, with fat men typically presented in much more forgiving and endearing ways, representations and narratives specifically about fat women (to be more specific, fat *white* women) are where the most explicit and complex narratives about fatness can be found on TV. For example, the "Blind Date" (1978) episode of *Taxi* (1978–1983) depicts Alex's romantic interest in Angela, a woman he talks to on a phone answering service. All of the characters in the taxi garage find her to be charming and funny, and thus encourage Alex to ask her out on a date. When Alex finally meets his date for the first time in person, she is not only a fat woman but also preemptively defensive about her body type because of past experiences of ridicule. Immediately after opening the door, she says to Alex, "I hate to disappoint you, but I'm Angela," and suggests, "we can stay here so no one can see us." The uncomfortable start to the date is exacerbated by Angela's constant self-deprecation in attempts of self-protection while Alex's friends (who crash the date) laugh at Angela simply for being a fat woman. Alex later apologizes to Angela for the circumstances surrounding their date and expresses his desire to know her better *despite* her fat body.

This episode is complicated because it demonstrates how difficult it is to be a fat woman, especially one dating in New York City, but it also suggests that at least part of the difficulty is Angela's fault for not believing that individuals may, in fact, be romantically interested despite or because of one's weight. "Blind Date" acknowledges she behaves defensively because of being judged and treated poorly in the past. Clearly, this feeds a cycle where she learns to defend herself against future hurt and rejection; but that very defensiveness creates other barriers to dating. However, preventing the episode from actually being empathetic or body positive is Alex saying upon the episode's conclusion that if he were a fat woman like Angela he "would not give up on love," but would instead "do stuff with my hair, wear makeup, go to the gym" to become more attractive. In other words, he wouldn't resign himself to despondency and defensiveness, he would *transform*. This episode of *Taxi* frames fatness as not inherently problematic, instead positioning the impact of fat stigma on intrapersonal thought and interpersonal interactions as the problem. However, fat individuals are not off the hook, so to speak, as they "choose" how to respond to the fat judgment and the scorn of others, either defensively like Angela or motivated to lose weight like Alex's hypothetical self-makeover.

One of the few television instances of critical discussion of fatness prior to the early 2000s is on *Designing Women* (1986–1993). The episode, "They Shoot Fat Women, Don't They?" (1989), begins by detailing Suzanne's anxiety to attend a class reunion because of her weight gain. The episode explores how difficult it is to find clothes as a fat woman (at one point Suzanne remarks, "You all act like I should order fabric from Georgia Tent and Awning!") and the classed dimensions of fatness (wealthy fat women shop at stores like "New Dimensions" while poor fat women shop at stores like "Fat Girls"). When Susanne wins the "Most Changed" award at her reunion due to her weight gain, it prompts her to give a speech about no longer caring what her classmates think about her body. She rejects the idea that "when you're fat, then you're supposed to be ashamed." Like *Taxi*, this episode of *Designing Women* discourages fat shame and fosters compassion for the experiences of fat individuals navigating a society that idealizes thinness. Yet despite rejecting fat shame, the show still positively frames Suzanne's lingering desire to lose weight.

Like the earlier examples in this chapter, fat embodiment as the impetus for adopting excessively strict diets is a common television trope, so much so that it remains the foundation of many contemporary weight-loss series articulated to discourses of the "obesity epidemic." In fact, narratives about dieting and weight loss are the most common ways in which fatness is overtly discussed on television, whether to prepare for social reunions like on *Designing Women*, *The Munsters* (1964–1966), and *Family Matters* (1989–1998) or in response to health concerns like on *The Fresh Prince of Bel-Air* (1990–1996). However, some television iterations of the dieting narrative reverse earlier representations of diets as over-the-top and unpleasant but ultimately necessary for love, health, or just living. These narratives position diets, not those who feel pressure to go on them, as the problem. These stories are some of the earliest examples of television expanding the possibilities of fat representation beyond reinforcing the importance of weight loss.

For instance, Roseanne and Dan commit to dieting together in a second season episode ("I'm Hungry," 1990) of *Roseanne* (1988–1997). Roseanne's inspiration to lose weight stems not from her own desire or bodily dissatisfaction, but from a beauty shop patron saying to her (while she is handing out donuts), "You have such a pretty face, it's a shame you keep it hidden under all that weight." Following the comment, Roseanne swears off junk food, but finds herself repeatedly triggered by food advertisements on television as well as the stash of cookies hidden in her family's kitchen cupboard. While restricting her caloric intake, Roseanne's whole world seems to revolve around the food she will not allow herself to eat, even "sneaking" food in the bathroom. Discussions throughout the episode bring up the double standards experienced by fat men and fat women, specifically that it is expected of men to gain weight while they age, but per Darlene,

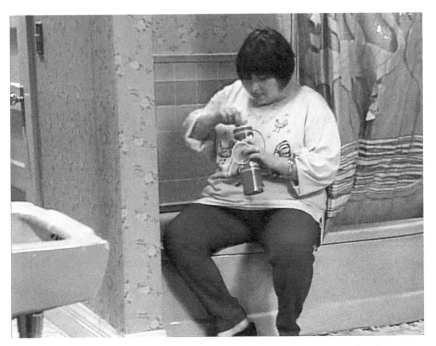

Figure 2   Roseanne straying from her diet on the "I'm Hungry" episode of *Roseanne* (1990)

"It doesn't look good on women." Eventually, Roseanne realizes the problem is not with her body; it's with both the people who shame her body and the diet itself. Although *Roseanne* features two fat individuals, the show rarely discusses fatness, and never points to the fat body itself as a source of comedy. This is likely the result of the fact that the creator and star of the show, Roseanne Barr, is well known for speaking out about fat rights, even writing a fat-positive autobiography in 1994.[26]

Twenty years after *Roseanne*, *Glee* (2009–2015) aired a similar episode, "Home" (2010), about a cheerleading coach instructing one of her cheerleaders, Mercedes, to begin an extremely low-calorie diet in order to lose ten pounds. Mercedes's attempt to eat a healthy lunch of chicken breast with salad proves to still be indulgent in comparison to another cheerleader's lunch of celery and Splenda. The episode is sprinkled with body-positive lines critical of excessive dieting, like Arnie saying, "You look beautiful no matter what. Diets don't work. As soon as you go off them you gain back the weight you lose." Eventually this borderline-starvation diet causes Mercedes to hallucinate that people are food and she passes out from hunger. By episode's end, Mercedes's body positivity is reinstated and a former cheerleader advises her, "You've always been at home in your body, don't let [the cheerleading coach] take that away from you."

Both *Roseanne* and *Glee* demonstrate in exaggerated and, strangely, not-very-exaggerated ways the complications, emotional effects, and even dangers of dieting by extreme caloric deficits. By the end of each episode both Mercedes and Rose-anne accept their bodies and reject the idea that they are somehow "less than" as large women. Their diets are at fault, not them. Similarly confident fat charac-ters who are rarely or never exhibited in relation to dieting or through fat jokes and stereotypes, but who visually contribute to body size diversity on the small screen, can be found across an increasing number of television texts, including Ellenor on *The Practice* (1997–2004), Donna on *Parks and Recreation* (2009–2015), Shirley on *Community* (2009–2015), Harriet on *Harry's Law* (2011–2012), Sookie on *Gilmore Girls* (2000–2007), Sadie on *Awkward* (2011–2016), Claudia on *Less Than Perfect* (2002–2006), and Miranda on BBC One on the United Kingdom's *Miranda* (2009–2015).

In addition to the way fatness is influenced by gender and sex, it is also con-nected to race generally and to stereotypes of Black women specifically. For example, *Beulah* (1950–1952), which is important for being the first television sit-com centering on a Black woman, also portrays "the ultimate example of the mammy." The mammy figure is typically a fat and desexualized mother figure whose central role is to serve white families.[27] In sitcoms of the 1970s and 1980s, elements of this fat Black identity lingered in representations of the "matriarch" on shows like *What's Happening!* (1976–1979), *Good Times* (1974–1979), and *The Jeffer-sons* (1975–1985).[28] Fatness and Blackness are again connected in another charac-ter trend on TV: the "bad" Black mother who is similarly fat but also "sassy," crude, and sexually aggressive. This particular representation extends back to *Amos and Andy* (1951–1953) and is present more contemporarily in shows like *The Parkers* (1999–2004).[29] Fat Black women on TV tend not to be connected to narra-tives of dieting or weight loss; instead fatness is contradictorily embedded in racialized or racist stereotypes of Black women as unruly or undisciplined.

It's important to consider multiple, intersectional aspects of identity and sys-tems of oppression when thinking about mediations of fatness. Representations of fatness through television's history are deeply influenced by gender, sex, race, ethnicity, and class; however, many of the representations and narratives about fatness in the vein of weight-loss shows privilege being *fat* as the primary and most important aspect of one's identity. Shows like *The Biggest Loser*, *Extreme Weight Loss*, and *My 600-lb Life* rarely discuss fatness in relation to gender, sex, race, ethnicity, or class, but that does not mean that gendered or racialized assumptions of fatness disappear when the shows are created or when we watch them.

These examples of fat representations and narratives throughout television's history demonstrate that contemporary ways of thinking about fatness have been present to different degrees for decades. Of course representations of fat-ness through the lens of weight loss were and are the most ubiquitous, but such stories and representations have never been as central to a show's premise or as intensely talked about as they are now. Today they are more overtly connected to health and medicalization, and to the resistance thereof. In fact, dozens of programs about fatness were developed across numerous channels in just the last few years, from reality shows about weight loss, such as *Shedding for the Wedding* (2011), to dramas that discuss fat issues, such as *Drop Dead Diva* (2009–2014), *This Is Us* (2016–), and *Dietland* (2018–). This trend is present not only in the United States but also on a global scale. Canada's *X-Weighted* (2006), Australia's *Big: Extreme Makeover* (2011), and the United Kingdom's *Supersize vs. Super-skinny* (2008–) are just a few examples of the fat TV created and circulated internationally.

A majority of fat-focused programs today reinforce dominant discourses of the "obesity epidemic"—that it's a health problem or even a medical disease—yet even within these televised stories of weight loss via exercise or surgery exist contradictions that create space for newer and less oppressive ways of thinking about the body. So while television, especially reality television, is often theoretically viewed as a reinforcer and extender of governmentality, which positions fatness as a problem in need of social and individual interventions or treatments in the context of the "obesity epidemic," this project instead focuses on the ways in which television about fatness regularly exposes its own incapacity to both fulfill this governing role and consistently support these disciplinary logics. Further, sometimes producers of television reject this role entirely, and instead explore different ways to think about fatness and bodies. Taken together, televised representations of fatness are thus full of both intrinsic and overt forms of resistance to dominant and disciplining fat narratives.

Why Television?

Television remains one of the primary ways many of us find both entertainment and information, and so much television is produced that some media critics claim we are in a period of "Peak TV" or a second "Golden Age" of television. However, arguments about the scope, reach, or popularity of one TV program or another are much more difficult to make in a post-network era of hundreds of channels and options to stream content on the internet or personal devices. During the network era, arguments for the importance of understanding television representations were easier to make because extremely large segments of the U.S. audience would be watching the same program at any given time. Watching the same television shows lent itself to a kind of common culture or shared experience among large groups of diverse people (although there is some debate as to whether this was ever the case, considering the historical lack of programs specifically or directly speaking to women or people of color). Because of this, TV scholars could understand the presence or popularity of particular representations as evidence of broader social or political trends, discussions, and negotiations. However, instead of television acting as a cultural forum like it was theorized in the network era, which emphasized the importance of TV because of its audience reach as a medium and role in the representation and negotiation of different ideologies, television in the post-network era produces multiple cultural forums, or an expanded forum, due to the multiplicity of content types available.[30] In this respect, individual series or channels may be less important than looking for particular representational trends across channels, platforms, and even television markets. Additionally, if we see particular kinds of representational politics emerge across multiple channels, especially ones targeting various demographics across different distribution platforms, television can still elucidate broader cultural, social, and political trends. In this way, television may be less of a synchronic cultural forum, in the sense that different ideologies or discourses may not always be in dialogue within the same text or at the same time, but may instead be an asynchronous cultural forum, where different ideologies or discourses, which are themselves already terrains of struggle, are encountered at different times, across multiple programs, channels, or distribution platforms. Furthermore, in addition to examining the interplay of different discourses on a given television series, I argue that we need to look at the inconsistencies, contradictions, and failures intrinsic to the discourses that are televised.

This project modifies theorizations of television, especially reality television, in relation to surveillance, governmentality, and the production of neoliberal citizens. Each discourse is already a terrain of struggle, and the complex and contradictory information circulating about health, fatness, and the body already negotiates numerous dichotomous notions, including agency and authority, public and private, and individualism and interventionism. These various discourses are further negotiated across television, which remains, and is perhaps even more so in the post-network era, a site of multidiscursivity. Even as TV may govern indirectly and circulate dominant discourses serving dominant social and political interests in the context of neoliberalism, it still negotiates and destabilizes those discourses in important ways. TV, then, exposes the limits of individualism and its own ability to effectively govern at a distance, or transform our bodies and behaviors, while it simultaneously weaves together and creates space for alternative, competing, and copresent notions of health, fatness, and the body. Thus, instead of television just reinforcing individualism and discipline in reflection of neoliberalism, television instead contradictorily disciplines and controls, while simultaneously exhibiting its own ineffectiveness to do either. Although television may, indeed, govern at a distance or act as a surveillance appendage (albeit an inconsistent one), it also operates as an asynchronous cultural forum weaving together various weight narratives and ways of thinking about fatness, health, and the body that can be generative instead of oppressive. Television is also a vehicle for medicalization, a way to generate capital for corporations, and yet, at times, it is a producer of programs that serve a kind of public interest or advance feminist narratives about body positivity. Thus, television (as a medium and as content) can be thought of in a variety of ways, all of which should be considered when analyzing television content, whether scripted or reality based, and the contexts enabling and constraining the types of content that are produced in the first place.

Despite the fact that reality TV exists not in a vacuum but as a part of a larger meaning-making system, a lot of reality TV scholarship still focuses primarily on the texts themselves as opposed to the social discourses circulating or contradicting each show's already incongruous messages. A majority of research on reality and makeover programming focuses on the way television replaces government and governs indirectly, at a distance, which means that both on-screen participants and audiences at home are encouraged to submit to surveillance in order to internalize self-monitoring and self-disciplining.[31] But much of the scholarship on reality or makeover television discussing governmentality and discipline on television does so without considering the polysemic nature of television and popular culture, even if the range of possible meanings or interpretations is limited. John Fiske argues representations contain as many contradictions as our social experiences,[32] and we need to incorporate this foundational understanding of TV to theorizing reality TV. Not all weight-loss reality shows offer the same steadfast messages of self-discipline, nor do audiences internalize only such messages; instead viewers often find themselves sympathizing, cheering for participants, sharing in their pride and disappointment, while also potentially ridiculing and blaming them for being fat. Further, the ways in which different TV series tell stories and create dramatic tensions problematize notions of self-discipline or self-control, surveillance, individualism, and the difficulty of changing or transforming oneself as much as these programs reinforce them. This is evident by contradictions within the weight-loss texts themselves (and texts as multiplatform meaning-making systems), the fact that these texts exist in a discursive terrain characterized by competing programs and discourses of health, medicalization, and body positivity or fat acceptance, and the numerous interpretations and reactions to these texts by viewers.

In response to an influx of reality television research focusing on surveillance, discipline, and governmentality, Dana Heller calls for us to look at the way reality TV, particularly makeover television, is dialectical and "marked by incessant border skirmishes over questions of elitism and populism, power and subordination, knowledge and exclusion, resistance and consent."[33] Heller outlines a more complex process that does not assume reality TV programs govern us and calls for scholars to look at contradictory messages within programs and the way people "talk back" to agents of governance or claims of expertise. Answering Heller's call, this project seeks to understand both how television attempts and fails to operate in terms of discipline and control and how television itself undermines and negotiates its own articulations to discourses of health and the medicalization of the body within the context of the "obesity epidemic."

Even though a considerable number of the fat television programs I look at are produced and exhibited in the United States, I also interrogate texts produced, distributed, and viewed internationally. Just as fat individuals exist everywhere, fat television can be found in most international markets as both U.S. programs are exported internationally and international programs are imported for U.S. audiences. The expectation that television programs should easily move across a range of markets is largely the result of the gradually deregulated and increasingly globalized nature of the television industry during the multichannel transition of the 1980s and 1990s. Although this project primarily tells the story of fat TV in the United States, in a world in which discourses often circulate internationally and industrial logics and practices operate with global audiences and markets (and policies) in mind, this project is inherently global in nature. For instance, dozens of countries have versions of *The Biggest Loser*, and numerous others are also producing and exporting original programing. Additionally, an increasing number of countries are also implementing regulations on television and advertising, especially children's television, because of the global scale of the "obesity epidemic." These global textual travels and international policy initiatives undoubtedly impact both the type of content produced in the United States and the way content takes shape in terms of representational and narrative choices.

Chapter Summaries

Chapter 2 provides an overview of the different discourses of fatness found across fat television programs in the context of the "obesity epidemic." I argue that televised representations of fatness primarily reflect one of three ways of thinking about the fat body: as a health issue connected to our personal choices, as medicalized and the disease of "obesity," and in terms of fat positivity and acceptance. These discourses of the body emphasize or downplay different ideas of fatness across television texts, regulatory policies, news articles, and academic journals, among other sources of entertainment and information. These discourses influence the way individuals make sense of and societies construct understandings of fatness, whether it should be celebrated or considered a problem in need of intervention or treatment, or whether it's a neutral type of embodiment or the result of poor lifestyle choices. How we view fatness has important implications for what types of interventions, treatments, or other solutions are considered necessary or appropriate, if any at all. Thus, this chapter works to provide an overview of the ways in which discourses of fatness are a terrain of struggle that reinforces power hierarchies and bodily dichotomies while emphasizing bodily struggles and resistance to oppressive ways of thinking about fat bodies.

Chapter 3 is devoted to exploring the ways in which television has established itself as a disciplinary and public service apparatus vis-à-vis dominant discourses of the "obesity epidemic." Citizens, public health officials, social scientists, and government regulators around the globe are increasingly interrogating or renewing their focus on the way television and advertising content is regulated, especially in regard to the impact of TV and advertising content on children, within the context of the "obesity epidemic." Meanwhile, the television industry employs several strategies to position itself both as acting within a kind of public interest and as a solution to the "obesity epidemic" instead of a cause. Television concern over the health and body size of television viewers is especially evident in relation to the cable channel BET and the BET Foundation's efforts to end "obesity" and children's television and its efforts to combat childhood "obesity," but it can be seen in different television texts and industry practices more generally around the world. This chapter thus demonstrates the way communication policies, or even just regulatory debates and regulator expressions of concern, continue to shape and constrain television industry practices as reported in trade and news publications, discussed in press releases, and found in various public service initiatives and television representations.

Chapters 4 and 5 explore the most prevalent form of fat TV, specifically weight-loss reality television, articulated to dominant discourse of fatness in the context of the "obesity epidemic." Programs like *The Biggest Loser* (2004–2016), *I Used to Be Fat* (2010–2014), *Heavy* (2011), and *Extreme Weight Loss* (2011–2015), among dozens of others, detail individual journeys of body transformation, or attempts at transformation, through expert interventions, changes in diet, and implementations of exercise routines. These programs, then, largely reflect dominant discourses of the "obesity epidemic" correlating body fat and health status, positioning both fatness and health as the result of our individual choices. More specifically, chapter 4 explores the way the "obesity epidemic" has become a "globesity epidemic" by examining the adoption of public health standards set by groups like the World Health Organization and perceptions that the United States is "exporting fatness." This chapter also looks at *The Biggest Loser* as an internationally circulated television series and the different national and regional format variations that simultaneously standardize increasingly global views of the fat body while undermining some of the most disciplining and shaming aspects of weight-loss series exported by the United States.

Chapter 5 primarily looks at the weight-loss series *Extreme Weight Loss*, *I Used to Be Fat*, and *Heavy*, as well as the ways in which these programs reinforce and contradict both reality television's surveilling and disciplinary role as well as dominant logics of the "obesity epidemic." These series are rife with disciplinary discrepancies in which televised weight-loss logics break down. By emphasizing tension, dramatic storytelling, and entertainment, weight-loss shows expose the inconsistences and inherent resistance within their messages of self-discipline, self-control, and transformation.

Chapter 6 considers another kind of fat television, namely programs representing fatness as a medicalized disease. These programs are part of a larger trend of medicalizing and pathologizing aspects of the body, positing that fatness is an embodiment in need of medical treatment as opposed to just a lifestyle change. Examples of medicalized television programming include *I Eat 33,000 Calories a Day* (2008) and, the focus of chapter 6, *My 600-lb Life* (2012–), which all visually represent the materiality, lived experiences, and medical statuses of those who are medically considered "super obese" or "morbidly obese." This chapter, then, explores medicalized television in relation to the medicalized fat body and how these programs offer inherent challenges to dominant discourses of fatness as a choice in the context of the "obesity epidemic," and how the labeling of fatness as a disease may mitigate disciplinary aspects of television spectacles while fostering fat sympathy as much as fat shame. While chapters 2 through 5 examine the ways in which individuals are encouraged to diet and exercise in order to lose weight, this chapter looks at the medical discourses and practices focusing on individual bodies without the same doses of individual blame in the contexts of hospitals, weight-loss clinics, and patients' homes.

Chapter 7 examines body positivity and fat-acceptance discourses across television texts like *Big Sexy* (2011), *Curvy Girls* (2011–2013), *Huge* (2010), *Mike & Molly* (2010–2016), and *Drop Dead Diva* (2009–2014). While there are still very few shows fully dedicated to explicit messages of fat positivity, fat bodies are becoming increasingly visible across the television landscape (without being linked to the same old dieting narratives) and more programs are embracing fat feminist politics. While the most overtly resistant examples are still far from common on TV, existing mostly across niche cable channels rather than on broadcast networks, their growing presence indicates both emerging industry lore and shifting social narratives of fatness that push back against the health and medicalized discourses of fatness in the context of the "obesity epidemic." Many of these programs generally avoid sustained discussions of weight loss and self-control, or surgery and disease, and actively work to represent fat characters and program participants as *actual* people as opposed to bodies in need of transformation.

A Note on Terminology

Throughout this project I use the term "fat" for specific reasons. According to Deborah Lupton, "in and of itself, fat has no meaning," but of course the word means different things to different groups of people.[34] The term "fat" has been reclaimed as a descriptor or type of body as opposed to an insult or derogatory term. I use the term to acknowledge that much like height, our weights naturally vary, resulting in some people having less body fat while others have more.

Further, I use the term "fat" in solidarity with the National Association to Advance Fat Acceptance and in accordance with the growing academic field of fat studies. In saying "fat," I also reject the terms "overweight" and "obese" as neutral body descriptors because of their health and medical connotations, which inherently position fat bodies as, at the very least, problematic. For example, a recent article in the medical journal *Clinical Cornerstone* calls for the classification of "obesity" as a disease in order to better treat the condition; "the condition" is defined as having a large waist circumference.[35] Additionally, the terms "overweight" and "obese" imply that an ideal or "normal" weight does exist and should be sought after. When I do use the terms "overweight" or "obese" throughout this project, it is because those are the ones used by the bloggers, journalists, researchers, or television programs I am referencing or citing, and knowing the specific terms being used is important for understanding what discourses are being articulated, not because I agree with the connotations those words have in regard to fatness or fat bodies. Please just imagine that there are scare quotes every time you see the words "overweight," "obesity," "globesity," and "obesity epidemic" throughout this book.

Finally, I do not intend this project to demonstrate that concerns over our bodies are entirely unwarranted or foolish, although I strongly believe that discourses and constructions of the "obesity epidemic" need to be scrutinized and challenged (and that the body mass index should be rejected as an indicator of one's health status). I am also not necessarily claiming that fat acceptance or critical biomedical claims are more accurate or true than health and medical research, nor am I trying to reveal some kind of "hidden truth" or "conspiracy" about fatness within the context of the "obesity epidemic." Rather, I'm concerned with how particular discourses of fatness in the context of "obesity epidemic" shape the kinds of television content we see, and thus how we broadly understand fatness. Although I do not see fatness as inherently unhealthy or as ugly or undesirable, I acknowledge that some individuals experience fatness as a health or medical problem. Others may dislike the appearance of fat on their bodies. Others may find their fatness to be physically impairing or socially disabling. Others still may be totally comfortable with or celebratory of their fatness. As a proponent of fat positivity and bodily *autonomy*, I'm not here to tell anyone what they should or should not do, what they should or should not think in regard to their own bodies. Instead, I am interested in the ways television shapes our understandings of fatness—as well as of our own bodies—and how interrogating representations of fatness can help us better understand television.

2   Competing Understandings of Fatness

Mike & Molly (2010–2016) debuted in the fall of 2010 on CBS, averaged between nine and eleven million viewers per episode, and became one of the most watched sitcoms on television throughout its run. However, several critics panned the show for its portrayal of two fat characters who meet at an overeaters anonymous group and start dating. One blogger for *Marie Claire* reacted to the pilot by saying, "I think I'd be grossed out if I had to watch two characters with rolls and rolls of fat kissing each other . . . because I'd be grossed out if I had to watch them doing anything."[1] This sizeist sentiment was not unique, as other critics of the show questioned whether it promoted obesity. For example, a *Fox News* article asked, "Should any of us be 'comfortable' with obesity? . . . Telling our children that weight doesn't matter because 'fat people fall in love, too,' is just wrong."[2] In addition to the TV commentators expressing concern over the representations exhibited on *Mike & Molly*, others were more ambivalent, praising the show for making fat bodies visible, but simultaneously condemning it for its frequent use of fat jokes and reliance on stereotypes.[3] These initial critical reactions to *Mike & Molly* demonstrate discursive tensions increasingly characteristic of the obesity epidemic, a time when fatness is simultaneously something to be abhorred, managed, treated, accepted, and even celebrated, all depending on whom you ask.

Debuting a few years later, in 2015, TLC's *My Big Fat Fabulous Life* (2015–) also navigates this contradictory bodily terrain. The show features Whitney Way Thore, who became internet famous after the virality of her YouTube video, "A Fat Girl Dancing." Way gained over one hundred pounds while in college due to polycystic ovarian syndrome. After years of struggling with eating disorders, depression, and low self-esteem connected to her weight, Thore became a proponent of body positivity and the creator of the No Body Shame Campaign. Through her YouTube videos and *My Big Fat Fabulous Life*, Thore works to counter assumptions that fat women are not physically active and that anyone should feel limited because their bodies are deemed "too fat," "too skinny," or "too broken." But while the show circulates messages of self-love, it also explores fatness as connected to disease, whether polycystic ovarian syndrome or other "obesity-related diseases" like diabetes, positioning weight loss as an important component of one's health. Because the show addresses both medicalized aspects of

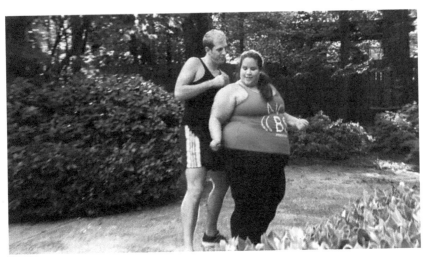

Figure 3   Whitney Way Thore and her partner practicing on the "A Fat Girl Dancing" episode of *My Big Fat Fabulous Life* (2015)

fatness and body positivity, *My Big Fat Fabulous Life* is concurrently and contradictorily accused of promoting obesity *and* condemned because Thore is perceived as not trying hard enough to lose weight.[4]

Both *Mike & Molly* and *My Big Fat Fabulous Life* act as sites for the convergence of ideas, images, and practices connected to different clusters of fat knowledge. Discourses of the obesity epidemic, which position fatness as a matter of global health, inform specific ways of talking about the fat body. Medicalized fatness, which positions fatness as a disease in need of treatment, similarly informs other ways of thinking, talking about, and treating the fat body. And the body positivity advanced by Thore as well as numerous other individuals, activists, and movements also inspires alternative thoughts about and practices associated with being fat. While *Mike & Molly* and *My Big Fat Fabulous Life* demonstrate the interplay of different sets of knowledge and practices, other fat-focused series on television are more dominantly articulated to just one discursive cluster.

In fact, most fat television shows are articulated to one of these three general ways of thinking about the fat body: as part of a global public health crisis, as a medical issue, and as a neutral or to-be-celebrated type of embodiment. These three sets of discourses are similar to the various frames of fatness discussed by Abigail Saguy, such as problem and blame frames, and the frames of fatness considered by Samantha Kwan and Jennifer Graves, such as beauty-fashion and health frames, but I instead look at how problem, blame, beauty, and health frames play supporting roles in these broader discursive clusters.[5] The particular frame used, or what ideas and details are both emphasized and deemphasized, across television texts, policy documents, and news media reports, influences the way individuals understand fatness, whether as something to celebrate or as a problem and has important implications for what types of interventions, treatments, or other solutions are considered necessary or appropriate, if any at all. Further, when these bodily frames are taken up by television, they contradictorily reflect and reinforce various discourses of the body while exposing the inconsistencies inherent in the discourses themselves, emphasizing television's continued role as a forum for storytelling, debate, and resistance as much as an effective discipliner at a distance.

Fatness as a Global Health Crisis

The most dominant discourse of fatness since the mid-1990s frames fat embodiment as a serious global health problem. In fact, the large influx of television shows encouraging weight loss, such as *The Biggest Loser* (2004–2016), *Extreme Weight Loss* (2011–2015), and *I Used to Be Fat* (2010–2014), is not surprising amid claims that, at least to some, obesity is this century's greatest public health threat. This idea is advanced by the U.S. Department of Health and Human Services and Department of Agriculture, which together publish nutritional recommendations in the guide "Dietary Guidelines for Americans," but also by the U.S. Centers for Disease Control and Prevention, governments across the globe, and the World Health Organization. News reports repeatedly detail the threat of obesity, to the point where the amount of fat on our bodies has become a concern of *epidemic* proportions. Beginning in the mid- to late 1990s, news reports became increasingly alarmist about obesity rates doubling over the last thirty years, with CNN reporting, "Americans are fatter than ever, and getting fatter!"

In fact, according to the CDC's 2017 "Adult Obesity Facts," a third of U.S. adults can be categorized as obese, with another third categorized as overweight based on the problematic body mass index.[6] However, the United States is not the only nation where citizens are labeled as possessing "dangerously" large bodies. The WHO reports 65 percent of all adults live in countries where body categorizations of overweight or obese are related to more deaths per year than body categorizations of underweight. According to their 2014 data, almost two billion adults twenty years of age or older are overweight, with six hundred million of those individuals considered obese. Naaru, Kuwait, Argentina, Egypt, Greece, Mexico, United Arab Emirates, and New Zealand all rank within the top twenty fattest countries in the world.[7]

Numerous studies hypothesize reasons behind this alleged global weight gain; some of the strangest include marriage, office snacking, clutter in the home, carbon dioxide levels, snooping, household chemicals, body shape wear, diet soda, and even just being a highly organized, emotional, and disciplined person. Yet the most regularly cited reason—also highlighted in connection to these other variables—is a lack of self-control, self-discipline, or personal responsibility. Studies consistently conclude that individuals who are considered obese demonstrate impaired self-control.[8] One such study finds a positive correlation between "evening chronotypes" and high BMIs, but argues that this relationship can be mitigated through—you guessed it—self-control.[9] Self-control is such a pervasive aspect of the obesity epidemic that if we generalize these conclusions to World Health Organization body categorizations, nearly two billion of us are considered to be lacking in self-control! Is it possible that citizens around the world collectively decided to shirk self-control in regard to their eating and exercise habits? Or if we go by data demonstrating that we are, indeed, becoming larger, is the explanation more complex than our personal lifestyle choices?

These associations between fatness and self-control—the fat body as the result of our personal choices—are important not just because of their pervasiveness, but also because they are deeply connected to assumptions about the personality traits and characteristics of fat individuals. One study finds, rather shockingly, that half of all obese patients are thought of as "awkward, ugly, and noncompliant" by physicians, while another third of obese patients are considered "weak, sloppy, and lazy."[10] Overall, most physicians attribute their patients' obesity to their personal behaviors.[11] Given these attitudes and assumptions, and numerous instances of fat shame and discrimination, it is no wonder fat individuals are less likely to go to the doctor.[12] Unfortunately, this attitude is present not just in the United States, as similar studies conducted in France, Australia, Israel, and the United Kingdom also reveal that physicians more commonly think of fat patients as lazy or lacking willpower in comparison to thin patients.[13] This attitude is also mutually reinforcing: our cultural ideas and associations between self-control and fatness are embedded in our medical, scientific, and scholarly understandings of fatness, and our understandings of fatness influence popularly circulated cultural ideas and associations. This only further stigmatizes fat bodies, legitimizes the importance of weight loss, and reinforces the connection between body size and health status (and social status too). Given all of this, it's unsurprising that citizens of the United States alone spend nineteen billion dollars a year on gym memberships and sixty billion dollars a year on weight-loss products and services.[14] Yet despite spending billions to prevent or try to reverse fatness, most of us remain fat.

These ways of thinking about fatness also dominate our news media. According to several analyses of U.S. news media, self-control—or the personal responsibility frame—is most commonly used when discussing the obesity epidemic, meaning that fatness is typically considered in terms of individual causes and solutions, such as individuals failing to balance the calories they take in versus the calories they burn through movement and daily bodily functions.[15] In fact, food selection and overeating are most often identified as the personal choices we make that may lead to the accumulation of extra adipose tissue,[16] followed closely by lamentations about our sedentary habits.[17] Basically, it is presumed we too often choose drive-through dinners and spend hours on the couch.

And like numerous other aspects of the obesity epidemic, this news emphasis on personal responsibility, or our individual lifestyle choices, is not limited to the United States. For example, a 2013 United Nations report ranks citizens of Kuwait, Saudi Arabia, Qatar, and Bahrain among the world's fattest. When a medical doctor in Dubai, United Arab Emirates, was asked to explain the high levels of body fat in the region, he replied, "A penchant for fast and fatty food and a lifestyle of late nights and no exercise. . . . Life gets easier but people tend to get busier and not take care of their own bodies."[18]

Discourses of personal responsibility have reached such a level of common sense, from the United States and United Kingdom to the United Arab Emirates, that alternative explanations for fatness, such as the lack of food regulation or farm subsidies encouraging the production and use of high fructose corn syrup or even proposed government and public health initiatives to "solve" obesity, are sometimes met with hostility. For example, a writer for the *Telegraph* argues in a piece under the headline "Fat People Only Have Themselves to Blame," "The more personal responsibility is removed from the direct relationship between eating and putting on weight, the more people can go on stuffing their faces, free of guilt—a crucial weapon for everyone in staying in OK shape." Even though this view can be considered extreme or polemic, it nevertheless demonstrates resistance to emerging, alternative narratives of the obesity epidemic that focus more on environmental, industrial, or genetic factors, demonstrating how interwoven the obesity epidemic and individualism have become. Emphases on individualism, whether self-control, personal responsibility, or lifestyle choices, which all fundamentally refer back to individuals being at fault, can also be found in U.S. government attempts to insulate different industries from blame for the obesity epidemic. For example, in 2004 the Bush administration started pushing back against World Health Organization guidelines for mitigating the obesity epidemic, which included various forms of government regulation. The Bush administration did not disagree with obesity being considered a major global health problem, but believed that instead of increased regulation, the government should emphasize and encourage personal responsibility among its citizenry.[19] Even after increased pressure from consumer groups to fight childhood obesity through policy, President Bush maintained, "It is an individual's responsibility to maintain a healthful diet, not the government's."[20]

While abdicating any responsibility for the obesity epidemic, government bodies also worked to repudiate any responsibility on behalf of the food industry, reemphasizing the supremacy of individual onus over the duties of industry and government. One hundred fifty bills were introduced across legislative chambers to insulate the food industry from liability, while reinforcing the centrality of personal responsibility in "fighting" the obesity epidemic. In 2004 and 2005, the U.S. House of Representatives tried to codify this idea into law when it passed the Personal Responsibility in Food Consumption Act, which earned the nickname "Cheeseburger Bill" in popular press reports. This bill prevented food marketers, advertisers, distributors, sellers, and numerous other roles within the food industry from being held liable for "claims of injury relating to a person's weight gain, obesity, or any health condition associated with weight gain or obesity." Although this bill did not pass a majority vote in the Senate in either 2004 or 2005, it inspired several successful attempts to insulate the food industry at the state level. In fact, twenty-five states passed "Cheeseburger Bills" or "Common-sense Consumption Acts" that prevent the food industry from implication in so-called obesity lawsuits.[21]

The logics of Cheeseburger Bills can also be found in several other governmental attempts pushing individuals to make lifestyle choices deemed personally responsible. For example, there are frequent calls to increase taxes, often referred to as "Twinkie Taxes," on the purchase of junk foods or sugary sodas, with seventeen states passing such legislation.[22] Even more extreme proposals to encourage self-control include fining fat individuals. Alabama now charges fat government employees twenty-five dollars more a month for insurance if they are not actively trying to lose weight, and former Arizona Governor Jan Brewer pushed for fat individuals to pay fifty dollars a year in fees for not meeting specific health or weight-loss goals. Other proposals include New Mexico's legislature debating whether to add a one percent tax to television sets and video game consoles (the tax would then fund an outdoor education program called "No Child Left Inside") and Mississippi debating banning fat diners from restaurants. Taking bodily punishment to its logical extreme, one writer polemically proposed *jailing* fat individuals as a "scare tactic" in a 2014 *Business Insider* article, saying, "Fat is an ideal menace to be targeted with a criminal law. To some extent, it's a subjective matter who is lazy or stupid, but it's pretty easy to figure out who's guilty of being fat. A law against fat would scare people into losing weight." Similarly, numerous states, including Texas, Pennsylvania, New York, and New Mexico, are now classifying childhood obesity as medical neglect, which can lead to the jailing of parents and limitations on custodial rights.[23]

Government actions encouraging personal responsibility through specific disciplinary actions or through taxes that punish the consumption of particular goods, which are framed as attempts to make it "easier" for people to be personally responsible, are not limited to the United States. The World Health Organization backed a report incentivizing farmers to sell healthy, fresh foods, while simultaneously encouraging tax increases on the purchase of "ultra-processed" foods.[24] The Tongan Ministry of Health is considering a "beefed up anti-fat tax."[25] Japan passed a law in 2008 setting maximum waist sizes for people over forty years of age.[26] At the same time, other countries are instead "incentivizing" weight loss as opposed to punishing fat embodiment. Dubai began giving people a gram of gold per kilogram of lost weight.[27] And in the United Kingdom, employers are encouraged (through potential government tax deductions and funding) to hold weight-loss competitions where individuals can earn money and other rewards.[28]

Despite rhetorically limiting government responsibility in addressing the obesity epidemic, numerous policies, initiatives, and practices simultaneously demonstrate continued government concern and action. However, government actions, initiatives, and interventions generally work toward fostering individual responsibility, balancing discourses of hands-off neoliberal ideology and the actual, pragmatic necessity of social support programs. This is evident across numerous city- and state-sponsored weight-loss initiatives encouraging individual action,[29] and various localized calls for banning certain foods in school cafeterias while sending "weight report cards" home to parents so they can individually monitor their children. Social programs emphasizing personal responsibility also parallel discussions of individual attitudes and behaviors dominant in public health campaigns. While various health organizations and groups do consider environmental, biological, cultural, and socioeconomic factors, it's usually to reduce or remove them as barriers to making individual choices and changes. Michelle Obama's Let's Move! campaign successfully convinced Walmart to lower the cost of fruits, vegetables, and whole grains by one billion dollars in 2011 (potentially providing greater access to low-income households) and funded "Play Streets" to create spaces in cities for families to play outside without worrying about traffic.[30] However, much of the campaign was about *encouraging* better nutritional labeling, *encouraging* schools to promote physical education, and *encouraging* individuals to make healthier choices by providing them with nutritional information through MyPlate. When systemic or broader issues—such as the role of the globalized food industry, the prevalence of high fructose corn syrup in most of our foods, and the potential impact of unwalkable suburbs, long commutes, and food deserts—are actually debated or addressed (as they are with aspects of Let's Move!), personal responsibility or individual lifestyle changes are typically maintained as the most important factor in one's level of body fat.

Despite the dominance of the personal responsibility discourses both within the United States and increasingly throughout the world, it is crucial to acknowledge that these logics frequently break down or prove ineffective. Decades of calls for individual lifestyle changes and personal responsibility do not seem to be affecting the obesity epidemic in any meaningful ways. If the obesity epidemic is, indeed, a problem in need of addressing, then focusing solely on the individual, and on the "calories in versus calories out" equation, does not seem to be achieving anything beyond producing and promoting individual shame and social stigma while letting food industries and governments off the hook. In an opinion piece for the *Guardian*, Ben Brooks argues as much, saying that the governmental and industrial emphases on individualism are akin to a "corporate defense strategy adapted from the tobacco and alcohol industries."[31] Besides, even if people do successfully lose weight by making individual changes to their diets or exercise habits, studies show the vast majority are unable to maintain that weight loss over long periods of time.[32] Some might say that regaining weight is also a sign of individuals lacking personal responsibility, but that is a similarly simplistic and unhelpful conclusion to a complex issue we are only just beginning to understand.

Medicalized Fatness

Another emerging way of thinking about fatness is as a disease, and this is reflected in television series like *My 600-lb Life* (2012–), *Inside Brookhaven Obesity Clinic* (2007–), and *Fat Doctor* (2011). On television, health considerations of fatness are connected to making different personal choices, whereas medicalized understandings of fatness as a disease are connected to treatments. These series typically depict individuals weighing upwards of four to six hundred pounds who "require" surgery or other kinds of medical intervention (hospitalization, psychiatry) to treat the fat body. While this way of thinking about fatness has existed concomitantly with health discourses of fatness for some time, only in the last few years has it emerged as a consistent alternative or addition to recommendations of diet, exercise, and other lifestyle changes.

Fatness was not a widespread medical concern throughout the early 1900s; instead, it was a source of cultural and social anxiety. In fact, these anxieties are what led to the development of the dieting or "reducing" industry, while medicine worked to *expose* dieting promises as false and unnecessary, typically arguing that fat was harmless and a sign of proper nutrition.[33] This skepticism and resistance to the weight-loss industry continued for decades, as is evident by a *New York Times* report in the 1950s about the American Medical Association declaring both that the U.S. obsession with dieting culture is a national neurosis and that dieting schemes do not have lasting effects on weight loss.[34] Some early weight-loss schemes included consuming Corpu-Lean's industrial toxin, dinitrophenol, to speed up the metabolism, ingesting tapeworms, and utilizing vibrating-belt machines to "slenderize" the body (versions of this are still sold today!). While these past weight-loss techniques may seem strange in retrospect, the diet industry actually has not evolved as much as we may think. As Pat Lyons points out, the dieting industry has been able to increase its presence and profits without showing any increase in effectiveness.[35]

Furthermore, dieting and fat-reduction techniques—whether emerging from weight-loss industries or, as argued by some, the field of medicine—are just as dangerous today and potentially more damaging to our otherwise healthy bodies and biological processes. Now people undergo invasive surgeries, take amphetamines, smoke cigarettes, drink diet soda, ingest cotton balls, eat only cabbage and grapefruit, or receive hormone injections to suppress the appetite.[36] Other proposed medical treatments include pills, such as Alli, that block the body's absorption of fat (one side effect: anal leakage), an external pump that removes contents from the stomach predigestion (referred to as a "tummy tap" in some popular press articles), and, of course, a wide variety of weight-loss surgeries from gastric bypass to gastric sleeves. Paradoxically, dieting to reduce body fat usually leads to the acquisition of more body fat over time, which continues to feed both the dieting industry and reliance on medical treatments to reduce fatness; all the while, dieting itself is linked to cardiovascular disease, stroke, diabetes, and impaired immune functioning.[37] Similarly, weight-loss surgeries are associated with serious side effects, including decreased metabolic syndrome, acid reflux, ulcers, bowel obstructions, and even fatal malnutrition.[38]

Just as strategies for fat reduction, whether originating in the dieting industry, the medical field, or some combination of the two, change over time, medical understandings of fatness have shifted in response to different contexts. When U.S. doctors began paying more attention to fatness in the latter half of the twentieth century, it was more common to consider extra adipose tissue a sign or symptom of something else rather than a problem itself.[39] As fatness became increasingly medicalized due to the development of weight-loss medications and surgeries, along with various scientific "discoveries" of genetic and hormonal components to weight gain and cozier relationships between dieting companies and medical practitioners, fatness itself became a type of embodiment requiring monitoring, treatment, and the label of *disease*. Of course classifying fat bodies as diseased is indicative of a broader trend toward medicalizing all conditions and aspects of the body.[40] From weight gain, sadness, bad breath, baldness, and the inability for some men to become erect when sexually aroused to normal functions of the body like puberty, pregnancy, or menopause, more aspects of being human are now under the purview of medicine. Correspondingly, according to Ray Moynihan and Alan Cassels, we are encouraged to take more medication for more illnesses or perceived illnesses than we ever have in human history.[41] And thanks to the Food and Drug Administration relaxing restrictions on marketing prescription drugs directly to consumers,[42] advertisements for surgical and pharmaceutical options proliferate across media platforms and are marketed in the same way as other banal consumer products and services. For example, a series of billboard advertisements across Southern California promised passersby, "Lose Weight with the Lap-Band! Safe 1 Hour, FDA Approved; 1-800-Get-Thin." These kinds of ads for weight-loss procedures coupled with the promise of insurance reimbursement likely contribute to the number of bariatric surgeries increasing each year.[43]

In 2013, the American Medical Association began *officially* referring to obesity as a disease, in addition to considering it a public health problem. While groups like the AMA, CDC, and WHO sometimes referred to obesity as a disease in the past, still implying that fatness is abnormal or a sign of the body functioning incorrectly, only recently has the impact of such a label been debated or purposefully used to denote a particular kind of ill health, one that is simultaneously considered a disease, a risk for disease, and a precursor to other diseases. The stated logics behind thinking about fatness as a disease are twofold. First, proponents of this label argue that it reduces the stigma and discrimination experienced by fat individuals by challenging the perception that fatness is simply due to over-eating or sedentary behavior.[44] If fatness is considered a disease, physicians may be less likely to think of their patients as weak, sloppy, lazy, and noncompliant, as would society at large. It's harder to fault someone for lacking self-control or personal responsibility when the individual's physical embodiment is diagnosed as a disease.[45] For example, the American Hospital Association argues that labeling fatness the chronic disease of obesity and "treating" fatness medically as well as behaviorally will mitigate assumptions that fatness is the result of a "character flaw."[46] This notion fits with studies showing when fatness is discussed in relation to factors beyond personality and individual behavior, such as genetics, biology, or the environment, attributions of blame or perceptions of lacking personal responsibility are reduced.[47]

Those arguing against the classification worry that defining one-third of Americans as diseased may actually increase fat stigmatization and reduce our sense of control over our own health (remember, health is considered a "choice"),[48] or encourage greater reliance on weight-loss medications and surgeries instead of traditionally recommended diet, exercise, and other lifestyle changes.[49] A recent study supports one of these points, finding that individuals are more likely to choose high-calorie foods after reading about fatness as a disease.[50] Furthermore, labeling fatness a disease can also be problematic for those who do not experience ill health as connected to having a fat body, meaning that this may strengthen as oppose to challenge automatic assumptions people make about bodily health based on a cursory visual "diagnosis."

The second reason the AMA explicitly labeled fatness a disease is to make it easier to treat obesity itself as well as "obesity-related diseases" like heart disease or type 2 diabetes. The AMA argues that insurance companies may be more likely to cover treatments, including bariatric surgery, if they are deemed to be medically necessary for treating disease. Insurance coverage would likely also encourage more people to undergo treatment. In this respect, some critics argue that the disease label is less about helping people and more about positioning fatness as a source of profit for pharmaceutical companies and those who perform bariatric surgeries.[51]

The labeling of fatness as a disease also gives greater influence on the topic to groups like the Centers for Disease Control and Prevention, which developed a Division of Nutrition, Physical Activity, and Obesity to research the causes and solutions to fatness. The CDC previously concerned itself only with infectious diseases, its original acronym standing for Communicable Diseases Center, so it's unsurprising that CDC materials about fatness use a medicalized and pathologized frame that talks about adipose tissue in terms of disease, infection, and transmission. This is evident even in their infamous "Obesity Trends among U.S. Adults" map, which uses BMI statistics to demonstrate how fatness "spreads" and rates increase, state by state, over several years.[52] Maps like these are commonly used throughout news broadcasts, obesity epidemic documentaries, and fat television shows to demonstrate the speed and severity of "spreading" fatness throughout the United States and the world, reinforcing the necessity of groups like the CDC for monitoring and treating fatness.

There are other ways in which we've thought about fatness as a disease or in relation to disease prior to it officially being categorized as such. The obesity vaccine currently being developed, commonly referred to as the "Flab Jab," will hypothetically inoculate people against gaining weight much like people inoculate themselves from chicken pox, tuberculosis, or influenza. Our interpersonal and social networks are also increasingly identified as important for understanding how fatness "spreads" from person to person. A 2007 *New York Times* article discussing the contagious aspects of fatness starts by saying, "Obesity can spread from person to person, much like a virus. . . . When a person gains weight, close friends tend to gain weight, too."[53] Evidence suggests individuals are 57 percent more likely to become obese if one of their friends becomes obese.[54] Even obesity epidemic rhetoric sometimes employs disease language in framing fatness as a public health threat. For instance, the rapid global "spread" of the disease of fatness is often linked to the proliferation of fast-food establishments "infecting" people across countries like Saudi Arabia, Egypt, Mexico, and China.[55]

Ultimately, while both the health discourses previously discussed and medicalized understandings of fatness as a disease position fat embodiment as a problem in need of a solution, they differ on the types of causes and solutions that are centered. Whereas health frames navigate a discursive terrain characterized by individualism in promotion of self-control and personal responsibility over the body, medicalization, on the other hand, positions fat bodies as diseased, as requiring medical monitoring and treatments like surgery or medication. In some ways, medicalized fatness as a disease does, indeed, undermine some of the commonly circulated discourses of self-control and personal responsibility as being both the root cause of and solution to fatness. The medicalization of fatness as a disease thus represents another narrative of obesity that shifts away from overemphasizing personal responsibility. But despite shifting the focus away from "diet and exercise," the emphasis is not shifted away from the imperative of losing weight. Instead, medicalized discourses of fatness suggest that fat individuals should undergo weight-loss surgery even if there are numerous, serious complications, including vomiting, dumping syndrome, and malnutrition,[56] or even if 50 percent of individuals regain weight within just two years after surgery despite continued restrictive eating practices.[57]

The medicalization of fatness and governmental attention to fatness as a global health problem position the body itself as an object of knowledge, one that legitimizes or normalizes particular kinds of bodies from which other bodies may deviate.[58] The normalization of these forms of knowledge by those in positions of power—whether political figures, regulators, medical doctors, public health experts or researchers—then creates and maintains a certain "[regime] of truth," which not only assumes the authority of "the truth," but actually "makes itself true."[59] In the context of the obesity epidemic, medical doctors and health researchers define, regulate, and surveil bodies, which purposefully differentiates between what bodies are considered "normal" (typically thin bodies) and what bodies are considered in need of expert intervention or treatment (typically fat bodies). According to Lauren Berlant, these conceptualizations and normalizations of health force living in particular ways, influencing whether we see our own bodies as "normal" or pathological or whether we diet, exercise, or turn to weight-loss pills or surgery to be considered "normal" instead of pathological.[60] While discourses of health and medicalization can be disciplining and oppressive, as Foucault reminds us, there is a "multiplicity of points of resistance . . . present everywhere in the power network."[61] Thus, we need to consider the way attempts to discipline our bodies through medicalization or as part of the obesity epidemic remain just that: attempts. These disciplinary strategies and efforts to force living in particular ways break down as much as they succeed; they prove themselves to be fallible as much as reliable. These increasingly normalized health and medicalized understandings of the body remain inherently contradictory and inconsistent, and they exist concomitantly with emerging and overtly resistant discourses of fat acceptance.

Fat Visibility, Body Positivity, and Fat Acceptance

The third way in which television represents fatness is through fat visibility, body positivity, and fat acceptance,[62] with shows existing on a continuum from intrinsic to overt forms of resistance to dominant discourses of the obesity epidemic. Television series reflecting these discourses range from the fat visibility found on *Mike & Molly* and *Crazy Ex-Girlfriend* (2015–) to the body positivity performed on *Girls* (2012–2017) or *Super Fun Night* (2013–2014) and the fat acceptance communicated on *Big Sexy* (2011). Fat visibility, body positivity, and fat acceptance all play important roles, although different and more or less radically resistant roles, in expanding the parameters for what is considered to be a "good" body or an acceptable body, to include *every* body. Although body positivity and fat acceptance include people of all genders and sexes, a lot of conversations center around women-identified individuals, making this discourse the most gendered of three discussed in this chapter. While representations of bodies of various sizes and shapes are increasingly common on television—although we still have a long way to go—characters and stories explicitly articulated to discourses of fat acceptance are only beginning to meaningfully emerge on television.

Discourses of fat acceptance push back against fat stereotypes and incessant reports of fatness as a threat to global health or as a disease in need of medical treatment. In news reports about the obesity epidemic, fat individuals are frequently shown eating "junk foods" (like the undoubtedly delicious nine-patty "T-Rex Burger" at Wendy's) and engaging in sedentary behavior (TV marathons on the couch). Fat individuals are more often depicted through isolated body parts and as lacking heads and faces.[63] Deborah Morrison Thomson refers to this as "spectacular decapitation." While this may protect the privacy of individuals featured on TV segments or in news articles, it also downplays or even eliminates their subjectivity and personhood.[64] Fat individuals are too often reduced to *being* their bodies, or only parts of their bodies, or are represented only through exaggerated embodiments of gluttony and laziness.

With news frames that perpetuate stereotypes, visual objectifications or "spectacular decapitations" of fat individuals, and the continuous release of seemingly dire statistics and reports framing fatness as a global health epidemic or medical disease, it comes as no surprise that size discrimination is prevalent. Studies show fat individuals have a more difficult time getting into top colleges, are subject to more severe harassment and stigmatization by their peers and teachers in school, and have a harder time finding housing or renting apartments in comparison to thin individuals.[65] Fat individuals also tend to be evaluated more negatively by their employers, are less likely to be promoted, and are generally paid less in the workplace than thin individuals.[66] The Citizens Medical Center in Houston, Texas, will not even hire applicants if they have a body mass index greater than thirty-five.[67] Airlines also discriminate against fat passengers.[68] The size and structure of desks in classrooms and lecture halls cause both physical and psychological pain as well as social shame for fat students.[69] Additionally, anti-fat bias is correlated to experiences of violence against women.[70] Fat women are ridiculed by police officers when reporting instances of rape or sexual assault (because fat women are perceived as "unlikely victims" due to their size).[71] There are many more ways in which fat individuals experience prejudice, discrimination, and violence because of the size of their bodies, and all of these examples support statistics documenting a 66 percent increase in the number of instances of weight discrimination in the United States over the past ten years.[72] Again, this is not a uniquely U.S. problem; similar instances of discrimination are reported in Australia, Mexico, and China.[73]

The fight against fat discrimination, stigmatization, and violence has roots in both the civil rights and feminist movements. The National Association to Advance Fat Acceptance has worked to improve the quality of life for fat individuals since the 1960s. Like other social and political protesters for justice and equal rights during that era, fat-acceptance activists worked toward ending fat oppression by holding "fat-ins" where they ate ice cream and burned diet books. A group calling themselves the Fat Underground criticized both the medical field and society at large for perpetuating a "genocide" against fat people while demanding that fat individuals be treated with respect in their publication "The Fat Liberation Manifesto."[74] Other groups formed or expanded their activism to include fatness as a political and social issue, including Girth and Mirth in San Francisco (1967) and the Iowa City Dykes (1972). During the same time period, the first books about fat pride and fat oppression were published, specifically Marvin Grosswirth's *Fat Pride: A Survival Handbook* (1971) and Susie Orbach's *Fat Is a Feminist Issue* (1978). These actions, groups, and publications demonstrate that both fat stigmatization and discrimination, including fat loathing, fat hatred, fat oppression, fat phobia, and weight prejudice, as well as resistance to such attitudes and practices, existed long before constructions of the obesity epidemic.[75] Even though fat resistance is far from new, it has expanded in scope and impact in parallel with intensified health and medical concern over the fat body. Today there is also the International Size Acceptance Association, the Association for Size Diversity, and fat-acceptance and activist groups in Canada, France, Germany, Spain, and Argentina. The existence of fat-acceptance groups around the world, while still small in overall membership numbers, demonstrates both increased prevalence of discourses of the obesity epidemic and explicit pushback against them.

Body positivity and fat-acceptance discourses were once relegated to small independent presses, such as the Iowa City Women's Press, which released some of the first fat-acceptance literature in the late 1970s, or alternative websites advocating coalition building and the development of fat-acceptance communities, such as the Rotund; today they are gaining more traction on popular (albeit still niche) online news and entertainment websites. Jezebel, xoJane, HelloGiggles, Bitch, Autostraddle, Everyday Feminism, Bust, and many more write body-positive stories with headlines like "9 Stunning Photos That Shatter Society's Stereotypes about the Perfect Body." Articles about body positivity and fat acceptance are also increasingly found across more mainstream news and culture sites, such as *Salon* and *Slate*, although they usually target fairly niche audiences under content categorizations like Style, Feminism, Women, or XX. The *Huffington Post* has a series of articles about body positivity and, at times, fat acceptance, with headlines like "Fourteen Painful Examples of Everyday Fat Shaming," "Why Thin Women Should Care about Fat Activism," and "Body Positivity Has No Size Limit."

Body-positive and fat-acceptance activists also maintain huge presences on social media sites like Instagram and Tumblr. For example, Virgie Tovar has almost thirty thousand followers on Instagram who are invested in her message of "Lose Hate Not Weight." Others create body-positive fitness spaces like Liberation

Barbell or blog about fat fashion in order to encourage readers to love and accept their bodies as they are, such as the Curvy Fashionista or Fat in the City. Some activists circulate zines, such as *Fat Girl* or *Fat Is Beautiful*, write books, such as Marilyn Wann's 1998 book *Fat!So?*, hold demonstrations outside of Victoria's Secret stores to protest mediated idealizations of thin women, create art that both celebrates fat bodies and challenges prejudicial ideas, and provocatively call for the conservation of fat individuals in the face of medical, governmental, and diet industry attempts to get people to—at least temporarily—lose weight. Other campaigns and body-positive projects include the Body Love Conference and the Adipositivity Project, which both push back against the notion that fat individuals should feel ashamed of their bodies or hide their bodies from view while centering alternative and expanded ideas of beauty not reliant on having a thin physique.

Though body positivity and fat acceptance already thrive on social media and across niche publications, they're gaining more attention and space in main-stream publications. For example, Lindy West started writing about feminism and fatness for Jezebel, but the popularity of her message led to a book deal exploring the topic, *Shrill: Notes from a Loud Woman* (2016), and to a column for the *Guardian*. The resonance of her messages led to an even bigger jump from being a columnist at a left-leaning, U.K.-based news organization to becoming a contributing op-ed writer for the largest (and one of the most respected) news-papers in the United States, the *New York Times*. This jump demonstrates that there are now larger and more receptive audiences for fat feminist activists and their messages. Or at least these ideas are provocative enough—without being considered too "out there"—to sell papers and digital subscriptions. Outside of West's column, the *New York Times* has also published op-eds questioning domi-nant obesity epidemic logics (through discussions of whether genes play a more significant role than our personal dietary choices in determining our weights) and asking why contemporary society seems to fundamentally and culturally fear fat.[76] In a similar vein, *Time* magazine featured a review of academic research showing overweight individuals actually have lower mortality rates than "nor-mal" weight individuals, which is contrary to the conventional wisdom of the obesity epidemic established and circulated by the CDC and WHO.[77] News headlines more frequently say, "People Can Be Fat yet Fit, Research Suggests," destabilizing assumptions that the presence of fat on one's body visually signifies poor health.[78] Articles such as these, which question or complicate dominant narratives, rarely occurred in national news platforms even a decade ago, but now are growing as commonplace as dominant frames of fatness as a health epidemic or disease.

Numerous actors and creators within the television industry are also reported to be embracing these messages of body positivity in rejection of the thin Hollywood ideal. Mindy of *The Mindy Project* (2012–2017), Hannah of *Girls* (2012–2017),

Donna of *Parks and Recreation* (2009–2015), and Sadie of *Awkward* (2011–2016) are all characters explicitly embracing the various shapes and sizes of their non-size-two bodies. A *New York Times* trend piece titled "Women on TV Step Off the Scale" explores this very notion by arguing the current generation of young women are more body positive after growing up with "after-school specials" about anorexia and Tyra Banks saying "So What?" as a retort to her weight-gain critics.[79] In fact, numerous celebrities not only are considering themselves "unapologetically not-thin," including singers Kelly Clarkson and Adele, but also, as with Lady Gaga, are part of a body revolution. Gaga even wrote on her own website after gaining twenty-five pounds, "Today I join the BODY REVO-LUTION. To Inspire Bravery. And BREED some mstherf**king COMPASSION." Responses to and interpretations of these particular celebrities' bodies vary, but the centering of these faces in the body-positive world demonstrates the way discourses of body positivity may still reinforce a limited range of body acceptability.

Overall, body-positivity and fat-acceptance proponents defy aesthetic ideals perpetuated by the fifty-billion-dollar U.S. beauty industry. Additionally, they challenge the medical and public health norms that are co-opted and circulated by the sixty-billion-dollar diet industry, which includes pharmaceutical companies, medical practitioners, and the manufacturers, marketers, and advertisers of diet products. These industries foster fat stigma and promote weight loss in order to "keep people dieting," or to continually convince individuals to undergo surgery, take diet pills, and join gyms, under the guise of health and the promise of beauty as opposed to actually helping people be healthy or feel beautiful.[80] Body positivity and fat acceptance, then, run counter to dominant industrial logics because they challenge beauty and "health" standards, while also demonstrating the ways in which those standards are mutually and erroneously reinforcing. Thin is considered to be healthy and beautiful, whereas fat is typically thought to be on the opposite end of both the beauty and health continuums.

Contributing to this, of course, is a media and advertising context that promotes a "culture of lack."[81] This culture positions individuals as needing to change themselves and their body sizes through self-discipline, willpower, and, most importantly, the purchase of certain products.[82] Women who are already accepting of their bodies, who already feel beautiful, or who focus on wellness and health as opposed to weight are not considered, at least superficially, a financially lucrative demographic for businesses relying on and reproducing the "culture of lack." People who resist, who adopt alternative ways of thinking, may be less likely to buy products to lose weight or conform to certain aesthetic ideals. However, emergent social discourses of body positivity and fat acceptance also exemplify the way empowerment can be commodified, leading some businesses and brands to co-opt messages of empowerment and body positivity to sell products as well as to create television programs relatable to audiences more in

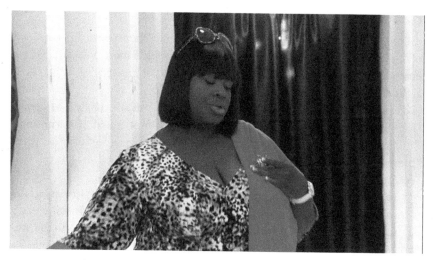

Figure 4   Donna Meagle from the "Pawnee Rangers" episode of *Parks and Recreation* (2011)

tune with body politics. For example, in 2005 Dove launched its "Real Beauty" campaign featuring "real" women (who wear clothing in sizes four to twelve as opposed to professional models sizes zero to four). The success of the Dove campaign spawned analogous campaigns by Nike, Special K, H&M, and designer Jean-Paul Gaultier. Even *Vogue* embraced body positivity in a photo spread featuring women of varying sizes, entitled "The Best Lingerie Comes in All Sizes." Nike's campaign depicts a "real" athletic and muscular women with copy reading, "My butt is big," "I have thunder thighs," and "My shoulders aren't dainty or proportional to my hips." The ad earned praise for turning the "taunts of high school boys" into sources of pride, but it received criticism for just reinforcing a different kind of bodily ideal. Special K's jump on the body-positive bandwagon is ironic considering it markets its cereals and breakfast bars as useful for weight loss. Like Dove and Nike, Special K began featuring "real" women in some of its advertisements and released videos of women talking about being "More Than a Number" (referencing both their pants size and weight) while encouraging women to "Shut Down Fat Talk." These advertising campaigns range from deeply flawed and contradictory to potentially empowering but still ripe for criticism. Yet, like numerous other advertising campaigns characterized by postfeminist discourses that position women primarily as consumers, all of them commodify empowerment and find ways to sell size liberation. Nevertheless, they all contribute to the spread of (limited) body positivity, which ultimately counters pervasive messages reinforcing the "cult of thinness" through products that are "light," "low," or "free," products that we are supposed to consume to become lighter and free from fatness.

Conclusion

Although body positivity is ripe for co-optation and often creates different kinds of bodily hierarchies, it creates an opening by which more radical ideas can emerge, and thus is not devoid of political and social importance. Whereas fat acceptance, which directly counters discourses of fatness as a global health crisis and medicalized as a disease, has greater potential to fundamentally alter oppressive ways of thinking about the body, it is less socially accepted. Unsurprisingly, this more radical view is met with considerable resistance and accusations that it "promotes obesity,"[83] glorifies a dangerous medical condition,[84] or just offers an "excuse" for fatness.[85] One critic of fat acceptance argues that shame is the best way to get people to lose weight, lamenting, "The stigma once rightly associated with obesity is disappearing as quickly as fat is accumulating."[86] Fat-acceptance detractors also label it a "threat to public health in a similar fashion to the anti-vaccination movement,"[87] and as damaging to society because it encourages individuals to make unhealthy lifestyle choices.[88] One op-ed in the *National Post* even goes as far as comparing fat acceptance to tobacco acceptance![89]

These kinds of claims and accusations—however hyperbolic and misinformed—present a challenge to emerging discourses of body positivity and fat acceptance, which individuals and movements counter in different ways. Some fat-acceptance activists or advocates navigate this discursive minefield by not entirely rejecting correlations between weight and health, but instead criticize those correlations when they are "exaggerated at the expense of shaming people, neglecting other aspects of health such as stress, sleep, mental health, and balanced eating."[90] Peggy Howell, the public relations director for the National Association to Advance Fat Acceptance, says they neither endorse unhealthy lifestyles nor encourage people to become fat, but are instead concerned with fighting fat discrimination. Howell adds, "As a citizen of the U.S., just because I carry more weight on my back doesn't mean I should have any fewer rights than anyone else."[91]

These compromises are undoubtedly frustrating to some who push for nothing less than full fat liberation from oppressive discourses of the body, but they can work as an important strategy for beginning these conversations and encouraging more people to embrace the body acceptance or body love mind-set. We need both radical proponents of body positivity and those frustratingly slow yet important incremental changes that can have a huge impact on deconstructing health and medical discourses of fatness. And television is an increasingly important space where those incremental changes can take place, whether intrinsically across weight-loss programs or overtly in series articulated to body positivity or fat acceptance.

3   *Does TV Make You Fat?*

TELEVISION AS CAUSING AND SOLVING
THE "OBESITY EPIDEMIC"

Television is regularly and simultaneously considered a destructive social and political force as well as a tool for education and the public good. Newton Minow famously lamented in his speech at the 1961 National Association of Broadcasters convention that television was nothing more than a "vast wasteland" (further downgrading the TV landscape to the status of a "toxic dump" in a 2001 op-ed for *USA Today*). This sentiment reflects both popular discourses denigrating TV, also evidenced by its 1960s nickname the "boob tube," and anxiety over the detrimental impact of mass communication on political and public life.[1] This anxiety is also evident in a 1988 PBS documentary, *The Promise of Television*, where commercial TV viewers are referred to as "consumers addicted to 'time-wasting' amusements."[2] Yet even before television became ubiquitous in American homes, many others viewed it as a "wellspring from which would flow great social, cultural, and intellectual benefits."[3] In this sense, TV became a potential educator and was frequently framed as both a tool for social benefit and a mechanism for shifting public opinion about international politics or racial politics and civil rights.[4] This dual, contradictory framing of TV, in terms of both critiques of content and discussions of television's positive potential, is important for establishing the way TV is currently vilified as a cause of obesity while also viewed as a solution to it. More specifically, popular assumptions about television watchers being couch potatoes with more sedentary lifestyles position TV as a culprit in our alleged global weight gain, inspiring both regulatory debate and certain media industry actions working to reposition television as a positive force or potential solution to a global health issue.

Even though few regulations on television *content* are actually implemented or enforced within the United States today, the significance of "regulation by raised eyebrow," which Thomas Streeter defines as "unfulfilled regulatory threats that cajole industry members into slight modifications," is necessary for understanding TV in the context of the obesity epidemic.[5] Some modifications include exhibiting more programming about weight loss, creating health campaigns and partnerships to reduce fatness, and changing advertising practices to prevent further governmental attention or metaphorical eyebrow raising. Both renewed regulatory attention and industry strategies and self-regulation reflect lingering notions of broadcast television's capability and, to some, responsibility of operating in the public interest. Whether the television industry *actually* acts in the public interest (it's fair to say that generally it does not) is not the focus of this chapter, which rather addresses how TV, both the medium generally and certain channels or programs specifically, is perceived to both contribute to and counteract the obesity epidemic through educational programming, awareness campaigns, and other television interventions.

Television practices, content, and regulatory debates in the context of the obesity epidemic recall the ways in which TV during the 1950s helped redefine the roles of and relationships between governments, citizens, and emerging "corporate citizens."[6] During that time, self-regulation came to define individuals, while notions of serving communities and volunteerism came to define corporate citizenship,[7] with television appointing itself to share in the responsibilities of educating and governing citizens. Today, some reality television is thought to represent a kind of return to this public service and educational tradition,[8] and although TV has replaced public affairs debates with "surveillance and voyeurism,"[9] emphases on personality responsibility, individualism, and choice have only intensified in the neoliberal era. And as this chapter demonstrates, when it comes to discourses of fatness as a lifestyle choice in the context of the obesity epidemic, television industries also still frame their actions and decisions in the tradition of corporate citizenship. Television thus continues to occupy a contradictory role and is framed by competing assumptions; it serves both a kind of public interest and the corporate interest of capital generation. It is both a tool for the public good and a source of social concern. TV can address fatness, but at the same time can allegedly make you fat.

Television Makes You Fat?

Paralleling TV's position as a tool for education or as a medium for public service is its long history of being denigrated for allegedly encouraging inactive or sedentary lifestyles. The first Zenith remote control in 1950 was called Lazy Bones. The expression "couch potato" is often levied against watchers of TV, with the average American viewing about five hours per day.[10] A 2004 article in *Broadcasting and Cable* jokes that perhaps we've even transitioned from "couch potato" to "couch burger, fries, and a shake" in the context of the obesity epidemic.[11] This particular television discourse is so dominant that the Malaysian government decided not to allow twenty-four-hour television transmission (choosing to instead shut down its four channels for a few hours each night) because of the belief that watching TV leads to obesity among viewers.[12]

With these expressions and fears circulating over television and its alleged effects on people, it comes as no surprise that TV is positioned as especially problematic in terms of children and fatness. News reports lament that children spend more time watching television than they do playing outside. For example, the *Irish Times* reported in 2007 that one in four Irish girls and one in five Irish boys between the ages of eight and twelve can be classified as overweight or obese according to the body mass index. The article then attributes these statistics to kids' increased likelihood of obesity if their mothers are obese and their increased likelihood of watching TV if their mothers do. Even though the article does not explicitly position TV as a factor in obesity, the connection is assumed to be common sense.[13] More evidence of the "commonsense status" of the "television makes you fat" discourse can be seen in numerous news articles, including one in the London newspaper the *Independent*, which states without any citation, "Sitting in front the television for multiple hours a day . . . is likely to make you fat."[14] Similarly, the *Vancouver Sun* reported in a 2011 issue, "Your television has an off switch and chances are if you don't use it, your children will grow up to be overweight or obese. . . . Simply turning the TV off makes children and adults more active."[15]

These examples reach the status of general knowledge or "common sense" with the help of numerous academic studies also positioning TV as a cause of fatness. In fact, according to one study, just owning a television in lower income countries, such as India, Bangladesh, and Zimbabwe, may quadruple your risk of obesity and diabetes.[16] Another study finds that metabolic rates are lower when individuals watch TV while lying down, and watching TV makes us more tempted to snack.[17] Research published in *Preventive Medicine* concludes, "Women, but not men, with higher levels of TV-viewing time had higher odds of reducing physical activity levels" and "abdominal obesity is associated with prospective reductions in physical activity."[18] Additionally, an article published in the *Journal of the American Medical Association* determines a positive correlation between time spent watching TV and a "risk" of obesity, leading researchers to recommend watching less TV as a method of obesity prevention.[19] Yet another study conducted by the Johns Hopkins University School of Medicine in conjunction with the CDC and National Institutes of Health finds that children, in particular, experience weight increases when television consumption increases.[20] Similar studies connecting children's "heavy television viewing" to an increased risk of being classified as overweight or obese have been replicated across multiple countries, including the United States, Mexico, and New Zealand.[21]

Much of this research relies on existing popular discourses in its assumptions and conclusions about the connection between television and fatness. For instance, an August 2012 article in *Physiology & Behavior* states, "While the causes of obesity are multifaceted, there is growing evidence that television viewing is a major contributor. Results of numerous studies indicate a direct association between time spent watching television and body weight. Possible explanations for this relationship include: 1) watching television acts as a sedentary replacement for physical activity; 2) food advertisements for nutrient-poor, high-calorie foods stimulate food intake; and 3) television viewing is associated with 'mindless' eating."[22] And one of the major conclusions from the article? "The simplest way to minimize the impact of television on the obesity epidemic is to watch less of it." Despite none of these studies being able to establish causation (that TV causes fatness), all of them inevitably prescribe watching less television in order to decrease the size of our bodies. Even through just these few examples, it's clear how these studies reflect and support popular discourses associating fatness and television. Beyond the scope of this project, however, is whether fatness and TV watching are actually related or whether watching TV causes fatness; rather, I establish the ways in which these kinds of television concerns and anxieties influence public opinion, activist campaigns, the proliferation of fat TV programming, health and regulatory debates, and, perhaps, media industry actions.

Television and the Public Interest

Throughout television's history, viewers have regularly been considered to be of low culture, lazy, or childlike.[23] Even regulatory institutions, such as the FCC, have during some periods adopted paternalistic positions toward TV viewers, usually infantilizing them and viewing them as homogenous masses in need of protection.[24] Even though most communication regulators no longer think, or ever *really* thought, that television's primary role is to serve the public interest or "protect" mass audiences allegedly in need of education and guidance, television policies and regulatory debates reflected such a view.

Television's role in serving the U.S. public interest extends back to the foundation of early radio broadcasting. Even though the form of early radio broadcasting in the United States was debated, specifically whether it would be a commercial or public system, defining the airwaves as public or comparing them to "public waterways" still influences the way we conceptualize television, even if only peripherally. Prior to the passing of the 1934 Communications Act, which established the Federal Communications Commission and primarily regulated radio, debates circulated over whether broadcasting as a commercial system could operate in the public interest in terms of providing educational or culturally uplifting programming.[25] The passage of the act settled the debate by answering in the affirmative that a commercial system could still consider the public interest and social welfare. This logic is also evident in the FCC being tasked by congress to not only regulate in support of developing the broadcast industry, but do so in a manner that "meets the informational needs of the public."[26] Interestingly, these decisions simultaneously downplay U.S. broadcasting's public interest role by favoring the adoption of a commercial system while connecting commercial television to it ideologically by "requiring" that broadcasters partially fulfill what nonprofit systems aspire to.

The development of broadcast television as a commercial system in the United States was unique, as most other countries had public broadcasting systems with the explicit goal of public service, meaning that they would be accessible and programs would be diverse, informational, and high quality. Public service television in Europe, according to Raymond Williams, took on a paternalistic role that had an explicit mandate of cultural uplift according to the standards, tastes, and values set by political, social, and economic elites.[27] Ien Ang states that television's noncommercial purpose was often viewed in terms of reforming the public or showing them how to "better perform democratic rights and duties."[28] Even though many of these public service systems have been replaced by commercial systems or exist concomitantly with commercial systems today, many public channels around the globe are still associated with similar public interest discourses.

The debate over what public interest or public service broadcasting actually means depends completely on whom you are asking. Robert McChesney partially defines public interest broadcasting as nonprofit and "aimed at providing a service to the entire population."[29] Conversely, according to Michael McCauley, industry rhetoric positions the public interest as government supporting a marketplace that fosters business or corporate growth and serves a variety of consumers.[30] Further, in the context of the obesity epidemic, not actively harming the public interest is positioned as analogous to serving the public interest. Regardless of how the public interest is actually defined, as industries most likely adopt the latter two definitions and frame their actions according to the former, discourses of the public interest have been circulated and debated as long as mass media have existed.

While broadcast TV is most often connected to notions of the public interest, debates over cable television's expansion throughout cities in the United States echoed similar concerns and goals. In 1972, the Federal Communications Commission stated that new cable systems "in the 100 largest television markets be required to provide channels for government, for educational purposes, and most importantly, for public access."[31] Even though the Supreme Court struck down this mandate in 1979, many cities and municipalities negotiating with cable systems were able to secure public access channels throughout the 1980s.[32] Additionally, the Cable Communications Policy Act of 1984 specifically encouraged the growth of cable systems in order to provide "the widest possible diversity of information sources and services to the public."[33] Even "must-carry" rules originally governing the relationships between local network affiliates and cable operators privilege access to information and the notion of the public interest. However, cable was framed with public interest goals more than it actually served them in practice. According to Patricia Aufderheide, rhetoric of the public interest was "universally invoked but rarely represented."[34]

For both broadcast and cable, appearing to act in the public interest, regardless of how it is actually defined, works toward framing the television industry as responsive to public concerns and helps them both evade government intervention and metaphorically lower the eyebrows of regulators. In fact, even during broadcasting industry deregulation in the 1980s, public interest standards were not rejected, just redefined: trusting the market is the best way to serve the public interest.[35] The FCC declared in its 1984 "Revision of Programming and Commercialization Policies" report, "Commercial television broadcasters will remain subject to an obligation to provide programming that is responsive to the issues confronting the community . . . it will be able to address issues by whatever program mix it believes is appropriate in order to be responsive to the needs of its community."[36]

While debates over the structure and control of television have been the primary focus of the FCC historically, public debates over content persisted despite being marginalized or without any real consequences.[37] Since the mid-1960s there has been a sustained effort to use regulation in order to change programming watched by children because of the effect content is believed to have specifically on them.[38] According to Heather Hendershot, "TV reformers see culture as something that is merely added onto an inherently innocent child. . . . Any writing on these youthful slates is potentially dangerous and potentially indelible."[39] These types of content concerns and debates often remain outside the purview of regulatory bodies, but these particular content debates corresponded with Newton Minow's "vast wasteland" speech, which emphasizes the broadcast industry's public responsibility to educate and enlighten viewers, and the FCC reorienting itself toward the regulation of content and serving the public interest. This example of public concern and regulatory response mirrors what is happening in terms of children's television and, more specifically, the junk food advertising that supports it. As early as 2004, reports in *Broadcasting and Cable* showed that television advertisers, in particular, were "getting slammed for promoting bad habits" by regulators and health officials.[40]

In the context of the obesity epidemic, however, debates concerning children's television and advertising are inspiring regulatory action both within and beyond the United States. Numerous groups call for the banning of "junk food" advertising during children's television programming, with one of the more recent calls in the United States coming from the American Academy of Pediatrics in 2011.[41] The logic underpinning this call can be seen in a study conducted by the University of Liverpool that connects viewing of commercials to children's appetites for sweet and high-fat foods.[42] These findings were then reported by a Singapore newspaper, the *Straits Times*, in 2011: "Television advertisements for junk food really do make children hunger for those treats, especially if they spend a lot of time watching television programs."[43]

This logic also supports South Korea's multistrategy campaign against the obesity epidemic. In 2010, the South Korean Ministry of Health, Welfare, and Family Affairs banned snack and fast-food advertisements during daytime television programming in order to restrict children's exposure to them. Interestingly, this ban does not specifically target children's programming, but instead includes all programming that children may have access to during the day. The *Korea Times* reports that the impetus behind this ban comes from increased warnings from experts of the "possible link between TV commercials encouraging consumption of these products and increasing child obesity."[44] Countries like South Korea may also be more eager to regulate advertising to children after research conducted by the University of Illinois showed Quebec's thirty-two-year ban on fast-food advertising correlating with teens living there being 38 percent less likely to buy fast food than teens in other parts of Canada. Additionally, it is estimated that Quebec kids consumed two to four billion fewer fast-food calories during that period than they would have without the advertising ban.[45]

These findings and their subsequent news reports, then, support numerous regulatory discussions and moves toward banning junk food advertising to kids and proposed or already established bans exist the world over. The World Health Organization's "Global Strategy on Diet, Physical Activity and Health" recommends limiting messages to children for "unhealthy" foods and encouraging the consumption of "healthy" foods, while also calling for a reduction in the total number of commercial advertisements for "junk food."[46] Other places seem to be following suit; for example, in Scotland, TV advertisements for any foods that are determined to be high in fat, sugar, or salt may be restricted until nine o'clock in the evening,[47] adding to a preexisting ban of "fatty food" advertisements during children's programming, "children" being defined as those under sixteen years of age.[48] Responding to reports that one-third of all U.K. children are classified as overweight or obese according to the body mass index, the United Kingdom became the first country to establish nutritional restrictions on advertising content directed toward children.[49]

Joining the United Kingdom, a number of other countries also regulate food advertising. France requires that healthy or balanced diet information must be provided along with any food advertising.[50] Nigeria and Thailand both require the government to approve advertisements for all foods. Australia and the Philippines both restrict "false advertising" in regard to the nutritional quality of foods. China, Denmark, Finland, and Malaysia all have regulations prohibiting snacks with low nutritional qualities from being advertised as meals and other regulations encouraging advertisements for balanced diets.[51] While there are still few examples of countries outright banning the advertising of "junk foods," it is consistently debated in Australia, Canada, and elsewhere.[52] These limited examples of international regulation are important because the U.S. television industry acts with the global in mind in terms of not only what kinds of programs are created (and where they are exported), but also the form programs take to potentially mitigate the growing global regulatory concern over television advertising and programming in relation to fatness.

Within the United States itself there is also a significant amount of regulatory debate concerning the relationship between obesity, particularly childhood obesity, and television viewing. For example, after Deborah Taylor Tate's appointment to the FCC in 2007, she set out to examine this very relationship.[53] Tate joined with FCC Chairman Kevin Martin and Sam Brownback, then senator of Kansas, in forming the Media and Childhood Obesity: Today and Tomorrow Task Force. This task force is composed of not only FCC members but also media insiders (including representatives from Disney, Discovery, Food Network, MTV, and Telemundo) and advertising and food executives.[54] The task force's goal, according to an article in Broadcasting and Cable, is to determine both "TV's Duty to Kids" and whether the food advertising industry and television channels are doing enough self-regulation to ward off further governmental attention.[55] Brownback spoke of its importance: "Judging by the sheer volume of media and advertising that children consume on a daily basis, and given alarming trends in childhood obesity, we're facing a public health problem that will only get worse unless we take action."[56] Of course, there are numerous government initiatives focusing on childhood obesity, including Michelle Obama's Let's Move! campaign, but this one is particularly important as it directly explores the relationship between television and health to the point where a governmental body is positioning television itself as having a role in the obesity epidemic. This provides further evidence that television is still partially considered in relation to notions of the public interest and its potential for both education and harm.

Currently, the Children's Television Act (CTA) of 1990 regulates broadcast networks, local affiliates, and cable operators in regard to advertising and children's programming. The FCC enforces limits on the amount of advertising that can air during children's programming (targeted to those under twelve years of age) to ten and a half minutes per hour on weekends and twelve minutes per hour on weekdays.[57] The FCC also limits "program-length commercials," which prohibits programs based on children's products or toys from advertising those products or toys during the show. Both Nickelodeon and ABC Family were fined one and a half million dollars in October 2004 for violating these limits.[58] While updates to the CTA include greater emphasis on and requirements for exhibiting educational programming, it has not (yet) been updated to restrict the kinds of food products advertised to children despite a few efforts. In 2004, a failed bill introduced by Senator Tom Harken (D-Iowa) proposed granting the Federal Trade Commission the ability to regulate advertising to children.[59] In 2011, the FTC, in conjunction with the Food and Drug Administration and the CDC released a report of suggestions, or "voluntary principles," on how food marketers and advertisers could respond to growing obesity epidemic concerns. Ultimately, the voluntary principles simply asked marketers and advertisers to encourage children to eat healthy foods, including fruits, vegetables, and lean meats, during thirty-second television spots and on-product packaging.

All of these regulatory examples and policy debates operate under the assumption that there are direct connections between what we see on TV and what we eat and do (they also operate on assumptions that fat embodiment is directly connected to what we watch, eat, and do). This model of media effects is discussed especially when it comes to children, who are positioned as more susceptible and impressionable, and thus in need of more protection. Regulatory discussions and policies evoking this media effects model also support the idea that television industry practices, in this case their relationship to advertisers, at least cannot be counter to the interests of the public, if not directly in the public interest. This further demonstrates television's contradictory status as a medium acting in the interests of both the public and corporations and as both a tool for the public good and a source of social concern.

Television's Own "Battle of the Bulge"

When actors within the television industry position themselves as responsible corporate citizens, they engage in a form of profitable self-regulation countering discourses both connecting and partially blaming TV for the obesity epidemic. This contributes to a long history of media industry self-regulation that aims to prevent actual government regulation. According to Heather Hendershot, "The free market approach to regulation assumes that self-regulation of content is adequate, inevitable, and benevolent because big business feels a sense of duty to consumers."[60] Furthermore, Anna McCarthy argues that the early broadcasting industry and corporate leaders positioned themselves as moral guardians over the interest of the nation.[61] This status is a strategy that encourages TV content to be seen as in the public interest, regardless of whether it actually is, and obfuscates the notion that exercises of corporate power may not *actually* be in the public interest.[62]

This public interest strategy combined with television's potential role in the obesity epidemic and the prevalence of fatness as a topic of concern encourage the development of programming appealing to large audiences. A 2010 article in the Australian newspaper the *Sunday Mail* explains that television programs dealing with fatness are popular with viewers because large numbers of people can relate to struggles over weight and can vicariously drop pounds through the people they see on the small screen.[63] One article in *Variety* argues that television networks have discovered that "big weight equals big business," while further elaborating, "with so many TV viewers struggling with their weight, showcasing more realistically sized people on reality TV would seem to be a no brainer."[64] Of course large audiences identifying with the weight issues exhibited on the small screen are also perfect for advertisers of diet plans, gym equipment, and health food. However, shifting the focus away from profit, *Variety* also reports that network executives and producers claim they are not trying to exploit fat individuals but are instead trying to inspire them, specifically quoting an executive producer of *The Biggest Loser*, Mark Koops, as saying, "This is an absolute epidemic and it's a real issue we're addressing."[65]

Additionally, *The Biggest Loser*, one of the foundational weight-loss programs, is evidence of the popularity and global success of fat television. The program features numerous contestants classified as obese who compete to lose the largest amount of weight for monetary prizes. Even though the obesity epidemic is often framed as a primarily Western phenomenon, the production of *The Biggest Loser* in twenty-five countries and regions demonstrates otherwise. Countries with formats of *The Biggest Loser* include Mexico (*¿Cuánto Quieres Perder?*; "How much do you want to lose?") and India (*Biggest Loser Jeetega*). Both countries are viewed by WHO standards as having high obesity rates, with India not far behind the United States,[66] and Mexico's rates surpassing those in the United States.[67] Even regions of the world that are generally not associated with fatness, such as countries in the Caribbean and those throughout Africa, may also become markets for fat television programming, evidenced further by news and health reports detailing the "problem" of obesity becoming as prevalent as the problem of malnutrition.[68] For example, the *New Zealand Herald* reports on rising obesity rates in Kenya in connection with a growing middle class and the opening of several Kentucky Fried Chicken restaurants. Several advertisements airing on Kenyan satellite television now advise people to watch their weights, when not long ago advice centered on encouraging parents to feed their children more food.[69]

Primarily Western countries and regions, namely the United States, the United Kingdom, Canada, Australia, and New Zealand, produce the bulk of fat television. Some programs mimic the competition format of *The Biggest Loser*, such as Australia's *Excess Baggage* (2012–) and the United Kingdom's *Lorraine Kelly's Big Fat Challenge* (2010–), but other programs focus on eliminating childhood obesity, food in relation to obesity and health, medicalizations of fatness in connection to disease and disability, or explorations of the obesity epidemic more generally. For example, ABC's *Shaq's Big Challenge* (2007) features former NBA player Shaquille O'Neal trying to help six "morbidly obese" children lose weight while simultaneously campaigning for mandatory physical education classes throughout Florida's public schools. The series aired only a few episodes but was notable for featuring Charlie Crist, then governor of Florida, which helped to weave narratives of both the personal responsibility of children and their parents as well as government responsibility within school systems as contributors to the overall health of children. Additionally, *Honey, We're Killing the Kids!* (2005–2007), a BBC series remade in the United States, imagines the futures of children if they continue to make poor dietary choices while spending too much time in front of screens. Each child is shown gaining weight in his or her computer-generated, hypothetical future, necessitating a health overhaul for the entire family. Both of these examples contrast with the notion of television as the cause of the obesity epidemic and instead show ways that programming can be interpreted as working toward a solution.

The television series *Jamie Oliver's Food Revolution* (2010–2011) aired in the United States, the United Kingdom, and Greece and serves as one of the best examples of television operating in a sense of the public interest. *JOFR* focuses primarily on the nutritional quality of school lunches (or lack thereof) and their impact on childhood obesity, but it also examines the problematic ways in which families eat at home. The show encouraged both school lunch programs and families to use fresh ingredients rather than processed and prepackaged foods. While *JOFR* was not very successful at "revolutionizing" school lunches due to resistance from public school officials, the show can be considered successful in terms of educating the public, or publicizing particular discourses, about the sad state of public school lunches and nutritional problems exacerbated by contemporary food regulations. For example, "pink slime" became a hot topic after Jamie Oliver demonstrated to a roomful of parents and primary school children how meat scraps are treated with ammonia and added to ground hamburger. Many credit this segment with popularizing the "pink slime" debates, as the segment received over a million YouTube hits and became an issue across numerous news programs and morning talk shows. Following this attention, multiple fast-food restaurants, including McDonald's, discontinued their use of the product as hamburger patty filler.[70]

Another example of the television industry producing programming framed both as responsive to the obesity epidemic and as operating in the public interest is HBO's *Weight of the Nation* (2012). For this documentary miniseries HBO partnered with several of the nation's leading public health groups and agencies, including the Institute of Medicine, the CDC, and the National Institutes of Health. The series explores socioeconomic and systemic factors contributing to fatness, the role of the food industry, and, of course, individual responsibilities for the size and health of our bodies. *Variety* highlighted the ultimate purpose of the documentary: "Like many HBO documentaries, this one seeks to inform, inspire, and perhaps even anger, rousing a citizenry from its complacency and unhealthy habits like drinking sugary beverages, from which average Americans derive nearly half their calories."[71] Furthermore, a producer of *Weight of the Nation*, John Hoffmann, states in a *Newsweek* article that the purpose of the program is to "sound the alarm" and motivate the nation to act.[72] These stated goals continue a long history of political and corporate leaders, as well as television creators, using documentaries to mobilize public opinion.[73] Regardless of whether these are HBO's actual goals in producing and exhibiting *Weight of the*

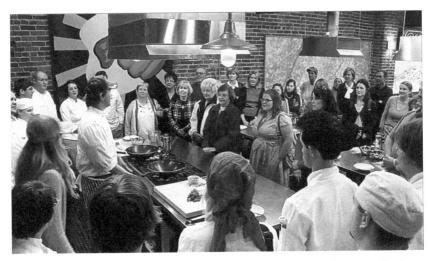

Figure 5   Jamie Oliver teaching West Virginians how to cook "healthy" foods on "Week 4" of *Jamie Oliver's Food Revolution* (2010)

Nation, the subject matter and tone of the documentary are perceived to be education and awareness squarely within the public interest tradition. Furthermore, twenty-minute *Weight of the Nation* episodes are also available for free on Amazon, iTunes, and other streaming services, framing HBO as being more concerned about getting information out to the public than keeping their content behind a profitable paywall.

Some television programs go beyond just engaging in issues of public interest and debate by actively encouraging their viewers to participate in certain activities. *The Biggest Loser* (at least in its earlier seasons) contains segments with healthy recipes for viewers to replicate at home, before directing viewers to websites for more health information or nutrition advice. This practice is fairly common on other health-focused shows that reach beyond topics of weight, such as *Dr. Oz* (2009–) and *The Talk* (2010–); however, the first season of *Extreme Weight Loss* goes one step further: encouraging viewers to exercise during commercial breaks. The show thus becomes a way, at least conceptually if not in practice, for viewers to squeeze in physical activity—almost twenty minutes of jumping jacks!—while being informed and potentially inspired by the content of the show itself. This commercial-break workout is similar to the "Couch Potato Workouts" frequently discussed and recommended on *Dr. Oz* and across lifestyle magazines, including *Cosmopolitan*, *Women's Health*, and *Prevention*.[74]

Beyond programming content encouraging diet, exercise, and weight loss, channels are working toward making their audiences "healthier" in other ways. One instance of this includes Discovery Fit and Health (formerly Discovery Health and FitTV) scheduling programs about physical fitness, including the

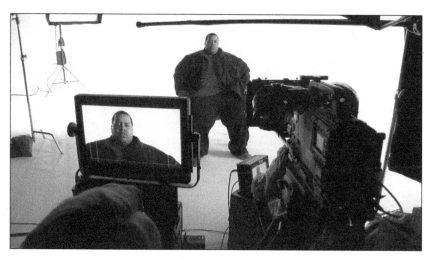

Figure 6   "Choices" episode of *Weight of the Nation* (2012)

BBC's *Are You Fitter Than a Pensioner?* (2010), which was retitled in the United States to *Are You Fitter Than a Senior?* (2011) because pensions are basically nonexistent. In this series, young, inactive kids with poor eating habits are paired with senior citizens at an active living community in California so they can learn the benefits of adopting disciplined and healthy lifestyles. Most of the channel's fitness and fat-fighting efforts can be found on its website, where blogs and videos provide viewers with everything from weight-loss tips to instructions for recovering from food poisoning. In addition to this content, the biggest Discovery Fit and Health initiative is its National Body Challenge. Beginning as a TV miniseries in 2005, the National Body Challenge became an annual event incorporating interactive online profiles, twenty-four-hour support and advice, customized meal plans, free thirty-day Bally Total Fitness memberships in many communities, and, of course, television programs featuring the weight-loss success stories of challenge participants.

The BBC aired a nine-part reality show, *Fat Nation: The Big Challenge* (2004), similar to the National Body Challenge, which "took over" a neighborhood in Birmingham, England. Fitness experts monitored neighborhood residents, taught them about nutrition and exercise, and set weekly weight-loss challenges and goals. Viewers at home were also encouraged to complete the weekly challenges and meet weekly goals, while the nation's progress was reported during each episode. Liz Cleaver, a representative of BBC Learning and Interactive, spoke about the impetus behind *Fat Nation* in a 2004 press release: "We know that lots of our viewers are worried about their weight and fitness and the health problems they could be storing up for the future. They want to do something about it, but the problem, as ever, is getting started. BBC Learning will take the sting out of it. We're going to help viewers to take that all-important first step and—crucially—keep it up." In writing about the debut of *Fat Nation*, the *Independent* reinforced the BBC's seemingly altruistic goals: "After decades of turning people into couch potatoes, it is to embark on an ambitious two-year campaign that is aimed at nothing less than reducing the collective weight of the British public."[75] Along with the show itself, *Fat Nation* includes interactive online services, such as tips to complete weekly challenges, personalized diet and health information, and a "personal locker area" where individuals can track their progress. "Sport Packs," including measuring cups for tracking calories and pedometers for measuring distances walked, were also sold. Of course part of the interactive service also included reminding viewers to watch the show.

BET, or Black Entertainment Television, is another channel working toward "bettering" the health of its viewers, but its efforts are simultaneously more comprehensive (in terms of content and brand partnerships) and targeted (in terms of audience specificity). In 2003, BET developed a foundation in partnership with the CDC to specifically address the health issues of greatest concern to its audience. Mostly, however, the foundation focuses on obesity because of U.S. Department of Health and Human Services estimates that 80 percent of Black women are classified as overweight or obese and Black women compose a large segment of the BET audience.[76] Furthermore, BET's audience is consistently labeled as especially "vulnerable" to the obesity epidemic, not only because of CDC body fat statistics but also because 2011 Nielsen statics reveal that African Americans watch more TV than any other constructed demographic group, averaging seven hours per day. This sentiment is expressed in a BET Foundation press release: "While the life expectancy and overall health of Americans has improved in recent years, the burden of illness and death in African American communities remains disproportionately high. We need to educate our community about the impact of some of our traditions and hopefully inspire them to change."[77] Thus, the combination of CDC obesity statistics and Nielson television watching statics necessitates, at least in the eyes of BET and the CDC, educational interventions to improve the "health" of BET's audience.

According to the CDC's website, "These community members depend on BET to not only bring them television entertainment, but to take the lead as a corporate citizen in providing them essential information and resources to address the social concerns and health needs of its community members."[78] The statement does a lot of work in framing BET's actions as within the public interest. By referring to audience members as "community members," it downplays their commercially defined status, and the labeling of BET as a corporate citizen emphasizes its outward-facing concern over civic matters. BET also emphasizes its civic role through several health campaigns and events held throughout the year. One campaign in partnership with General Mills, referred to as A Healthy

BET, seeks to reduce obesity rates, particularly among Black women. In order to accomplish its goal, A Healthy BET produced public service announcements for exhibition between series, held seminars and public forums in a few cities throughout the United States, and created fitness challenges, programming segments, a dedicated website, a toll-free health hotline, and other brochures and information to educate BET viewers.[79]

An example of BET incorporating BET Foundation practices into its programming can be seen in its music video countdown show, *106 & Park* (2000–2014). The point of this segment, according to the hosts of the show, is to increase awareness among Black audiences that fatness is, indeed, a "problem." This framing of "awareness" as a solution seems to presume that Black individuals somehow evade exposure to the deluge of obesity epidemic news reporting and that variations in body norms, specifically that Black women may be more satisfied with their body sizes overall,[80] need to change in order to comport with medical and governmental recommendations. In one episode of *106 & Park*, Asher Roth (who is, interestingly, white and rather slender) raps to raise obesity awareness: "Question: what are we feeding the kids? Man, they keep getting bigger like obesity is. Creeping up on us with each McDonald's, how wide are we going to let our pants legs get? It's kind of good because I like fat chicks, but I feel bad watching the fat kids with their double chins flapping and underarm skin wiggling when clapping. . . . Nothing is possible without good health." Even though this rap is offensive for a number of reasons, the hosts of *106 & Park* praise Roth for caring enough to intervene in such a "serious health issue" within Black communities.

Other rappers testify to the importance of raising awareness and education on BET as well. Before debuting his new music video, Fat Joe took the opportunity to inform BET viewers about his weight-loss journey: "I wasn't educated. A doctor never approached us and told us we needed to change. We didn't realize we could be twenty-seven and have a heart attack. That's why we are trying to spread the knowledge right now. I am just a person who ate right and exercised. Get healthy, lose weight, save lives." Both of these examples, which are characteristic of other BET segments about fatness, also operate under several assumptions: one, individuals are unaware that certain actions or habits may be unhealthy; two, if individuals do become aware, they will want to change; three, fat bodies can simply be transformed through better personal choices and behavioral changes; four, individuals should want to change their "unhealthy" behaviors and transform their fat bodies; and five, there is a direct connection between body size and health status.

Many attempts to change personal behavior through these kinds of awareness-raising or interventionist educations rely on the theory of reasoned action, which, according to Kathleen LeBesco, assumes that "behavior intention is the immediate determinant of behavior and that all other factors that influence behavior are mediated through intention."[81] However, knowledge that a particular food is "bad" does not automatically change our attitudes about it nor our long-term consumption of it. These notions that education or awareness will lead to behavior change fail to account for the complexity of human behavior and assume that knowledge about something should directly alter individual actions despite potential competing desires, needs, or impulses.[82] This logic ultimately puts responsibility for health or weight loss into the hands of newly "enlightened" or "educated" individuals.

In addition to incorporating discussions of fatness into small segments, BET aired the special *Heart of the City: Dying to Eat in Jackson* (2009). This special tracks how the "killer" of obesity has been passed down from generation to generation in the city of Jackson, Mississippi, except here there is a switch from educating people about the consequences of their personal choices to blaming community and generational traditions, namely soul food and consumption of fried foods at church gatherings, for the high rates of obesity among Black individuals.

Adding to personal choice failings and problematic food traditions is also the idea that fat and body acceptance within Black communities is a major contributor to higher rates of obesity. This notion reflects popular discourses that frame Black women, in particular, as being problematically complicit in their own fatness and unable—or unwilling—to "help" themselves. In November 2009, BET held a roundtable, "The U.S. Obesity Epidemic: African Americans at Risk," featuring health journalists and medical experts. One expert on the panel, Dr. William Gibbs, medical director of the Department of Rehabilitation Medicine and founder of the Pediatric Healthy Lifestyle Program at New York Hospital, argues that issues of weight perception and lack of cultural stigma are major problems in need of addressing by public health experts. As his evidence, Gibbs shares an anecdote about one of his patients saying that she did not "know she was obese until he told her that she was . . . she didn't realize there were certain body parameters where one's health is in jeopardy." Another panelist echoed a similar sentiment: "There is almost a reverse distortion of body image, thicker women fighting weight loss and slender women wanting to gain weight. This may account for the staggering statistic that four out of five African American women are overweight or obese. And what's most alarming is that these women are making a choice to live at an unhealthy weight." These expressions of concern over Black women's bodies are rooted in a long history of scholarship arguing that Black women are more likely to both reject idealizations of slenderness and view beauty as less connected to weight in comparison to white women.[83] According to Andrea Shaw, African diaspora cultures have historically resisted notions of slenderness as an "ideal state of embodiment," instead favoring "robust female bodies."[84] Shaw contends that fat Black bodies can primarily be viewed as resistant to the gendered and racialized ideals of the West that ideologically erase Blackness and fatness in exchange for a kind of mainstream aesthetic "acceptability." These notions popularly circulate and influence industry practices, as evidenced by both BET's campaign and *The Biggest Loser* regularly citing fat tolerance in Black communities as a contributor to the obesity epidemic.[85]

Therefore, Black individuals are positioned not necessarily as at "fault" for fatness, but as influenced by cultures and traditions that allegedly give preference to larger bodies and "a taste for fried food."[86] This then frames certain cultural beliefs, practices, and traditions as problematic and as occurring at a "cost." Black women, in particular, are understood to underestimate the size and shape of their bodies,[87] which may cause them to "deny health problems."[88] These "costs" are also reinforced in numerous academic health studies. For example, the National Institutes of Health: Heart, Lung, and Blood Institute views Black women's generally positive attitude toward healthy, full-figured bodies as both troubling and a barrier to weight loss.[89] The American Diabetes Association, through its weight-management group Shaping America's Health, and the Obesity Society (a scientific society for the study of obesity) released a joint statement pointing to variations in behavior and culture by ethnicity and race as detrimentally impacting obesity rates. The statement also notes that Black individuals idealize larger body sizes, express less body dissatisfaction, and have food traditions that increase the risk of obesity in children who are also exposed to more food advertising on television.[90] Similarly, another study links increased sedentary activity (including TV watching!) to low-income, particularly African American, families.[91] Just as panels, studies, and statements like these continue to identify different patterns in food consumption or physical activity, they also tend to conflate cultural, racial, ethnic, and even geographic factors that shape our identities when we should instead, at least according to medical anthropologist Alexandra A. Brewis, "think in more theoretically informed ways about how and why poverty, ethnicity, minority status, and so on coalesce to create obesity risk."[92]

Ultimately, certain "populations," namely Black women, are viewed as not making "educated" personal choices about what to eat or how to feel about their own bodies. While some weight-loss programs, such as *The Biggest Loser* or *I Used to Be Fat*, regularly position fatness as a moral failing or the result of laziness, BET and the BET Foundation resist those types of messages as they are inexplicably linked to long-standing racialized and racist discourses of Black individuals within the United States. For instance, researchers find that discussions of fatness in relation to race repeatedly parallel narratives of the "welfare queen" that position Black individuals as irresponsible "drains on public resources."[93] Furthermore, Abigail Saguy contends that fatness is differently framed throughout news media when intersecting with particular races and classes. She finds that a "white, wealthy anorexic girl" is usually considered a victim to illness outside of parental control, while a "black, poor, obese boy" is considered to have a health problem that "may be the result of parental neglect."[94] Deborah Lupton makes a similar claim to Saguy based on relevant research: "Mothers of non-white ethnic or racial groups are positioned as particularly neglectful in allowing their children to become fat, and it is assumed that such mothers require special education so that they can more effectively perform their responsibilities in monitoring their children's weight."[95]

BET thus frames its audience as in need of awareness and education about the impact of individual, parental, and cultural food choices and traditions or norms regarding body size preferences. In this sense, BET's actions somehow fit with Shaw's understanding of fat Black women not necessarily being incapable of complying with body ideals, but instead as being unwilling to comply or as indifferent to those ideals. But while Shaw views these acts of "chosen disobedience" and "disruptive behavior" as expressing a "lack of desire to ingest the alien ideologies that have already rendered her beyond the periphery of dominant culture,"[96] BET and public health interventions assert that if only they can convince Black women that these behaviors and attitudes are actually detrimental to their health, they may be persuaded to change. This assumed ignorance, of course, is also insulting, but allows BET to frame itself as a corporate citizen looking out for the health of its audience as opposed to capitalizing on obesity epidemic concerns and our collective bodily anxieties the way other channels may be. Further, BET's non-TV health interventions do advocate community involvement and individual empowerment, particularly localized public forums, fitness challenges, and cooking classes, which have the potential to more productively tap into the health concerns of individuals not automatically related to the physical size of their bodies. However, BET's television-based emphasis on awareness and education, framed as an altruistic television industry intervention, and the assumptions about the interconnections between fatness, health status, racial or ethnic identity, and cultural practices remove from possibility individuals accepting their bodies and striving to be happy or healthy across a spectrum of sizes.

Problematically, the other major television audience segment experiencing a similar level of obesity epidemic intervention to Black women is children, reflecting the regulatory attention and policies discussed earlier in this chapter. In accordance with public interest and social concern discourses still framing television, reform groups have long been concerned about television's impact on children's physical and mental health.[97] In the United States, children spend almost twice as many hours watching television as they do in the classroom by the time they graduate high school,[98] 25 percent of children's food consumption is estimated to occur while they are watching TV,[99] and children with televisions in their bedrooms tend to get less sleep, thus becoming more obese.[100] The group Active Health Kids Canada even laments that advocating for healthy diets will not work well if kids continue watching two to four hours of television per day.[101] Findings like these undoubtedly inspired the American Academy of Pediatrics to release a policy statement, titled "Children, Adolescents, Obesity, and the Media," that relays concern over the way food advertisements increase children's desires for junk foods, how staying up late to watch TV may limit sleep, and how children have far too much daily screen time. The policy state-ment further reads, "American society couldn't do a worse job at the moment of keeping children fit and healthy—too much TV, too many food ads, not enough exercise, and not enough sleep."[102]

As a result, media industry actions consistently attempt to mitigate these concerns, whether through the 1952 television code developed by the National Association of Radio and Television Broadcasters to affirm the industry's respon-sibility to children viewers or the American Association of Advertising Agencies' creation of the Children's Advertising Review Agency (CARU) to self-regulate advertising content. By monitoring and censoring children's television in the past, networks hoped to quell fears, reduce complaints, and maintain their "benev-olent image" as corporate citizens.[103] In fact, even during deregulatory periods, children's standards departments were retained by cable channels because the industry lore was that the public "would not tolerate unregulated children's pro-gramming."[104] This public relations move, which demonstrates even cable chan-nels framing themselves as operating in or at least considering the public inter-est, is particularly important as only broadcast networks traditionally rely on standards and practices departments to review and potentially modify content transmitted over public airwaves. However, specific concerns over the vulnera-bility of children to televised images led many cable channels primarily targeting children, such as the Cartoon Network, to develop their own internal standards departments.

Growing concerns over childhood obesity in the early 2000s not only renewed public calls for the FTC and FCC to restrict junk food advertising to kids, but also provided a much more persuasive reason for doing so in comparison to earlier health concerns like tooth decay.[105] This concern likely provided the impetus for the National Association of Broadcasters to collaborate with the U.S. Depart-ment of Health and Human Services and the Ad Council in order create and distribute public service announcements for the 2005 Childhood Obesity Preven-tion Campaign. A few years later, the National Association of Broadcasters also approved a resolution to fight childhood obesity by supporting Michelle Obama's Let's Move! campaign. NAB's initiative included helping "inform and educate our nation's children and parents on the benefits of healthy eating and living" and coordinating a "Flash Workout" between member stations around the coun-try and local schools.

Television channels are also invested in creating content that appears to counter childhood obesity in order to prevent not only content regulation and appease concerned parents,[106] but also advertiser regulation, especially consider-ing food advertisers spend upward of three billion dollars on TV marketing annually.[107] In fact, Dan Jeffe, executive vice president of the Association of National Advertisers, argues that *food* advertising essentially keeps children's programming on the air.[108] By spearheading their own anti-obesity initiatives or committing a percentage of their nonprogrammed airtime to health messages,[109] channels hope to show government regulators they are doing enough (or more than enough) to protect their advertisers (who are a major source of revenue) and themselves from actual government interference. An article in *Broadcasting and Cable* sums up the whole situation nicely: "Like a kid caught with a hand in the cookie jar, networks and advertisers are red-faced with guilt, even as they beg viewers and Washington not to punish them. After all, they live off the fat of the land."[110]

Yet television executives still frame their actions as less about generating capital and safeguarding their advertisers and more about protecting children. A Nickelodeon spokesperson, Dan Martinsen, reiterates industry concern over children's well-being: "This is something we have to do, not from fear of government crackdowns, but because kids programmers are obligated to safeguard their impressionable and vulnerable audience."[111] Nickelodeon's president, Nick Zarghami, offers a similar sentiment: "We're doing a lot of work helping kids understand the value of a healthier lifestyle and exercise."[112] Additionally, a Cartoon Network executive, Stuart Snyder, states, "Childhood obesity is an epidemic to our country, and that's why for the past three years we've done the 'Move It Movement Tour,' which is all about getting kids to eat healthier and to exercise more and to live a healthier lifestyle."[113]

Mirroring prominent policy debates in terms of both problems and solutions to the obesity epidemic and correlations between obesity and television watching, a significant amount of children's television content now encourages physical activity, which directly counters discourses of TV as being unhealthy and a sedentary activity, and demonstrates industry responsiveness to widespread social concern over childhood obesity. Disney's *JoJo's Circus* (2003–2007), PBS's *Poobah* (2003–), and Nickelodeon's *Dora the Explorer* (2000–2015), among others, encourage kids to get off the couch and move around or dance as they are watching.[114] This trend is present not just in the United States, but all over the globe. A similar children's program, *LazyTown* (2004–2014), produced in both the United States and Iceland and airing in over one hundred countries, urges kids to choose physically active, healthy lifestyles.[115] Nick Jr. in the United Kingdom also exhibits a once-a-week program, referred to as "Toddlerobics," that is essentially an exercise class "designed to improve children's co-ordination, concentration, bone and muscle strength."[116]

Several Canadian programs also specifically encourage kids to be physically active both while watching TV and throughout other parts of the day. The increase in these types of programs is a response to findings indicating that 91 percent of Canadian children do not get enough exercise.[117] In anticipation of reports encouraging people to turn off their children's televisions in order to reduce rates of youth inactivity, TV turned itself into a fitness activity. TV Ontario's *I Dare You* (2006–2008) challenges children to engage in three physical exercises during the program. Other shows, such as Treehouse TV's *Roll Play* (2006–) and *4 Square* (1996–2007), feature segments asking viewers to mimic the dances and actions depicted on the screen. The children's program *Bo on the Go!* (2007), produced by DHS Halifax and aired by the Canadian Broadcasting Company, also encourages physical activity, broadcasts in seven different countries, and has been translated into multiple languages.[118] These examples directly contradict the sedentary, couch potato discourse often associated with television, which is especially important to the television industry within the context of the obesity epidemic. When messages circulating in the popular press urge people to turn *off* the TV and be active,[119] these programs demonstrate that individuals should instead turn *on* the TV to be active.

Physical activity is not the only element of health circulated by both dominant obesity epidemic discourses and contemporary children's television; healthy eating practices are also increasingly addressed. For instance, *Sesame Street's* (1969–) Cookie Monster learns in a 2005 episode that cookies are "sometimes food," engaging directly with concerns over children's diets and childhood obesity while careful to advocate for food variety and moderation as opposed to traditional notions of dieting (especially commercial diets intended for adults). The Cookie Monster moment marks a foray into children's programming becoming more conscious of health messages in accordance with growing public, governmental, and medical concern. However, Cookie Monster including vegetables in his daily diet is not an isolated incident on *Sesame Street* but rather one part of a wider initiative on the show called "Healthy Habits for Healthy Life." This initiative encourages kids to increase their physical activity while teaching them about the importance of eating vegetables through a multilanguage multimedia kit for families with tips on how to eat healthy foods on a budget.[120]

Beyond exhibiting content encouraging physical activity and other "healthy habits," the television industry is employing several other strategies that work to mitigate correlations between television watching and high rates of obesity. Instead of creating fitness programs, channels may opt for entirely stopping transmission during certain parts of the day. One instance of this practice is Nickelodeon New Zealand no longer playing its usual Sunday cartoon lineup for two hours. Instead, the channel airs automated, rotating segments featuring games and physical activities.[121] This is particularly interesting as it prevents Nickelodeon from receiving advertising revenue during that two-hour period, making the practice appear especially altruistic and establishing that the television industry's business imperatives are not out of sync with public concerns.

Advertisers themselves are also self-regulating and pushing more "kid-friendly" diets. For example, Kraft Foods announced in 2005 that it would limit the kinds of advertisements placed during television shows aimed at children. Lunchables and Oreo commercials were largely suspended, and the Kool-Aid Man began focusing more on the promotion of sugar-free versions of Kool-Aid instead of the sugar-heavy original. A Kraft spokesperson, Mark Berlind, explains these changes as recognition of parental concern over the impact of advertisements on children. Of course this frames even the food industry as being amenable to issues concerning the obesity epidemic, although not so amenable as to stop using cartoon characters on product packaging.[122]

In an even bigger attempt to appear responsive to obesity epidemic concerns, Disney independently decided not to air "junk food" commercials during any of its programs to demonstrate its efforts to "combat childhood obesity."[123] In determining what foods are considered "junk foods," Disney established its own nutritional guidelines, specifying that it would allow advertisements for breakfast cereals only if those cereals contain fewer than one hundred thirty calories and ten grams of sugar per serving.[124] Items that meet the Disney nutritional standards will get the "Micky Check," akin to the American Heart Association's logo on food products signaling to consumers that they are allegedly "Heart Healthy" food options.[125] Of course this form of self-regulation is quite self-serving. The practice frames Disney as concerned about the public interest and the welfare of children, which is particularly important amid debates concerning government regulation of "junk food" advertising around the globe. In fact, the European Union released a white paper in 2005 warning the food industry to either make changes to the way food is advertised to children or face legislation forcing them to make the necessary changes. The EU health and consumer affairs commissioner, Markos Kyprianou, explains, "The signs from the industry are very encouraging, very positive. But if this doesn't produce satisfactory results, we will proceed to legislation. I would like to see the industry not advertising directly to children any more."[126] Thus, if content producers like Disney as well as food advertisers like Kraft demonstrate self-regulation (even if according to their own arbitrary nutritional guidelines), then the raised eyebrows and regulatory debates about restricting advertising and TV content can be deemed unnecessary.

Conclusion

In addition to television industry attempts to demonstrate that television content and advertisements supporting the creation and exhibition of that content are operating with the public interest and with the health and well-being of individuals in mind, TV industry executives and advertisers are also shifting criticism toward the U.S. government, arguing that while industry regulation is not the answer, industry self-regulation alone cannot be a solution to obesity. For example, Dan Jaffe points out the contradiction between expressions of government concern and government inaction, arguing that while industries are spending billions on education and healthy foods marketing, governments continue to cut physical education and nutrition education programs from schools.[127] Jaffe expresses similar dismay—whether real or feigned—in a 2005 opinion piece published by *Broadcasting and Cable*: "But what concerns me most is that, despite all of this positive and progressive action, the advertising industry continues to be targeted as a leading contributor of this epidemic." This sentiment seems to suggest that while television executives are fine with benefiting from TV being framed in terms of corporate citizenship, or with TV being a discipliner at a distance and tool for education and social awareness, there are limits to what media companies will take on and the amount of criticism they're willing to endure.

As long as discourses of the obesity epidemic circulate, fat television texts will continue to be distributed and exhibited, especially with the potential profit that can be gained from large audiences around the world both identifying with the subject matter and finding the topic to be personally relevant. In this sense, fat television clearly operates in the commercial interest. But beyond the obvious imperative of profit is what these particular programs and channel actions achieve during a time when the advertisements that fund television, and television itself, are frequently cited as a reason for fatness in the first place. TV channel anti-obesity initiatives and educational content, industry self-regulation in response to regulatory raised eyebrows, and actual policies regulating advertising to children internationally are based, first, on the premise that TV has effects, and those effects are harmful. However, if television itself appears to mitigate those harmful effects, as fat television texts and children's programs that encourage physical activity do, then there is no further need to regulate the industry, as it is already operating with the public's interest in mind and will have a positive impact. In the midst of fatness being considered a dire social concern, popular discourses connecting television to fatness, especially TV watched by children and other constructed populations deemed "vulnerable" by health experts, are gaining enough traction to warrant government debate or regulation and industry action. While the former attempts to fix the problem caused by this possible correlation, the latter aims to prove that this connection no longer stands and maybe never did. Ultimately, the influence of policy debates and the concerns of regulators and television maintaining its status as a corporate citizen serving the public interest in the context of the obesity epidemic demonstrate television's continued contradictory framings as an entertainer, educator, and discipliner at a distance.

4   *The Globesity Epidemic*

ADAPTING WEIGHT-LOSS TELEVISION
AROUND THE WORLD

The 2012 opening of the first KFC location in Nairobi, Kenya, produced a lot of both local excitement and international concern. The opening was viewed by some as Kenya "catching up to the rest of the world," further evidenced by a growing middle class and increased consumer spending, but others believed the impact of fast-food consumption would prove detrimental to Kenyans' health. Economic growth is transitioning Kenya, like other sub-Saharan African countries, from experiencing a hunger crisis to an obesity "problem." In fact, 40 percent of Kenyans living in urban areas are considered overweight, while another 15 percent are considered obese, according to the World Health Organization's (WHO) categorizations.[1] Similar statistics can be found in Nigeria and Botswana, with one in eight men in Nigeria and more than half of all Botswanian women categorized as obese. Other developing countries outside of Africa, including India, Singapore, and Malaysia, are also simultaneously dealing with malnourishment and high rates of obesity.[2] The prevalence of obesity in all these countries exemplifies why Lauren Berlant, among others, refers to fatness as, perhaps paradoxically, "a predicament of privilege and of poverty."[3] "Fat is no longer just a developed world problem," according to Ian Birrell, a journalist for the *Guardian*. "Today more people in poorer countries go to bed each night having consumed too many calories than go to bed hungry."[4] The inclusion of countries like Kenya and Malaysia that many would not suspect as being part of the obesity epidemic demonstrates why fatness is now framed as an issue of global concern, or a globesity epidemic.

Constructions of the globesity epidemic make weight-loss reality television relevant to numerous national and regional television markets. *The Biggest Loser* (2004–2016), a foundational weight-loss television program airing for seventeen seasons, is syndicated in over ninety countries and has expanded to formats in twenty-eight different countries, including Australia, Brazil, Mexico, South Africa, Ukraine, Turkey, Latvia, Brunei, the Philippines, and the Netherlands. There are also regional variations, such as *The Biggest Loser Asia* (2009–2010) and *The Biggest Winner* or *Ar-Rabeh El-Akabar* (2006–2009), and iterations in Russia and Indonesia. In addition to *The Biggest Loser* format, weight-loss programs exist across numerous countries, such as Canada's *X-Weighted* (2006–) and Australia's *Big: Extreme Makeover* (2011), which both follow similar narrative structures but instead focus on the personal journeys of just a few participants. And, of course, there are several U.S. variations on a theme, including MTV's *I Used to Be Fat* (2010–2014), A&E's *Heavy* (2011), and ABC's *Extreme Weight Loss* (2011–2015), which I will discuss in the next chapter. Even though these shows reflect location-influenced understandings of fatness and frame fat individuals in slightly different ways, all of these programs fundamentally reinforce dominant discourses of obesity where fatness is a health problem deeply intertwined with individualized notions of personal responsibility, self-discipline, and self-control.

This chapter first discusses the ways in which fatness became understood as a globesity epidemic, a neologism used to indicate the spread of fatness around the world, paralleling the global spread of reality weight-loss television even in countries like Kenya and Malaysia. International TV producers create and import content based on their knowledge of and assumptions about local audiences as well as "imaginary connections that bind together different segments of the public both within and beyond the nation-state."[5] The globesity epidemic acts as one such binder that frames large and seemingly disparate groups of people through the same weight-loss lens. The global proliferation of weight-loss television further evinces the transnational mobility of makeover television,[6] and the "global currency" of "(neo)liberal models of selfhood and citizenship."[7] According to one producer of *The Biggest Loser Asia*, certain topics just have "mass appeal" on television, such as "singing, dancing, sports, *weight* [emphasis added]. . . . [These are] relevant issues to every age, demographic, and culture."[8] Issues like the obesity epidemic are thus thought to easily transcend different cultures and nations, likely achieving this status as concern over fatness became global in scale.

While the weight-loss premise does flow fairly easily around the world, the process of adapting U.S. content to other countries and cultures typically results in downplaying some of the most individualized, dramatized, and competitive aspects of *The Biggest Loser* format, exposing them as a specifically "American vision of contemporary selfhood."[9] The examples of format changes discussed throughout this chapter, although still reinforcing weight loss as desirable or necessary, resist and at times contradict the disciplinary logics of weight-loss reality television in the United States.

Constructions of the Globesity Epidemic

While fatness has long been considered to negatively reflect on the self,[10] the amount of fat on our bodies is also now positioned as being detrimental to humanity on a much broader scale. Popular culture reflects these anxieties as exemplified by the film *Wall-E* (2008), where fatness is shown to literally be the destroyer of human civilization. Fatness is positioned as less of an issue of appearance, preference, or status, although it still remains all of these things, but is instead considered "a matter of life and death."[11] For example, an advisory panel for the 2010 Dietary Guidelines for Americans declared obesity to be this century's greatest public health threat,[12] and the U.S. Department of Agriculture considers obesity to be the foremost U.S. nutritional problem. The World Cancer Research Fund considers obesity to be a top *global* health threat.[13] Others believe fatness will deplete the world's natural resources as our collective weight constitutes "242 million extra people of normal weight," and those bodies take more energy to live and move.[14] Additionally, the International Obesity Task Force argues that obesity is an "international scourge" resulting from a lack of willpower,[15] which will overwhelm medical systems around the world.[16]

Although the United States is typically thought of as the fattest country in the world, it is usually ranked somewhere in the top ten or top twenty, depending on the list. Fiji, Samoa, Kuwait, Saudi Arabia, Chile, Argentina, Egypt, Mexico, and Jordan all have similar rates to the United States, and most of Europe is just behind the United States according to the WHO.[17] Albania, Armenia, Algeria, and Lesotho all actually have higher rates of childhood obesity than the United States, which ranks twentieth overall.[18] Even though the United States does not have the highest rates of obesity, it is regularly positioned as the source of spreading fatness. For example, it's argued that China's obesity problem is the result of food marketers successfully convincing Chinese consumers to join Americans in their fattening snack habits.[19] *Arab News* reported in 2002 that the 52 percent obesity rate among adults in Saudi Arabia is the result of Saudi citizens embracing the "trash of American culture," becoming "victims of the cruelest aspects of globalization."[20] This sentiment is also expressed by the U.K. series *Supersize vs. Superskinny* (2008–), which refers to the United States as the "Fat Fatherland" and as being on the "frontlines" of the obesity epidemic. The show also sends its participants to the United States in order for them to witness the health problems experienced by those categorized as super morbidly obese (as if the United Kingdom is not home to similarly categorized people).

The United States is now considered by many to be exporting obesity around the world, with some labeling it "America's Deadliest Export."[21] A 2013 article in the *Week* explains, "The U.S. is fueling the 'globesity' epidemic by exporting the worst of its eating and exercise habits to once-healthy foreign cultures."[22] An article in *Medical Daily* echoes the same sentiment: "America may also be sending the world its obesity epidemic as others in developing nations adopt first-world eating and exercise habits."[23] For example, Qatar is now seeing "shocking levels of obesity" due to "radical lifestyle change" attributed to higher levels of wealth and globalization, to the point where "cars have replaced camels and fast food and home deliveries take the place of home cooking."[24] However, others rightly point out that the U.S. role in the globesity epidemic is less about exporting individual behaviors and more about the impact of U.S. trade policies and the fact that it is home to global food manufacturers that create and distribute high-sugar and high-fat processed foods around the world. Researchers argue that high rates of obesity in Mexico are the result of high U.S. tariffs on sugar and subsidies for corn production, which lead to the overproduction of cheap high-fructose corn syrup used in countless products both consumed in the United States and exported to Mexico.[25] When food marketers in the United States did not know what to do with high-fat "turkey tails" in the 1950s, they began exporting them to one of the country's trading partners, Samoa. They quickly became a delicacy there, replacing leaner traditional food options like fish and leading some to identify them as a cause of climbing obesity rates in Samoa during the 1960s.[26] Today, 80 percent of Samoans are categorized as overweight or obese.

These increasingly globalized influences and understandings of fatness are deeply connected to international nongovernmental organizations like WHO. The first WHO discussion of obesity took place in 1997, and by the next year it began referring to obesity as a "public health crisis of the greatest magnitude."[27] In 2000, WHO released a report titled "Obesity: Preventing and Managing a Global Epidemic," which the International Association for the Study of Obesity (IASO) views as a turning point in widespread governmental adoption of the WHO's views on fatness as "the biggest unrecognized public health problem in the world."[28] Prior to global standardization of weight metrics by the WHO, different systems to categorize people were used within and across countries. Throughout the 1980s and 1990s, the U.S. Departments of Agriculture and Health and Human Services defined being overweight as between 24.9 and 27.1 on the body mass index (BMI).[29] During the same time period, the National Institutes of Health differently classified men as overweight when above a 27.8, women when about a 27.3.[30] Even though many nation-states now use BMI, others believe it to be a problematic measurement of body fat levels, overall health, or both. For example, in the United States, BMI is the primary metric for categorizing bodies and for implicitly determining individuals' health status, but in Canada health policy reflects skepticism over BMI as a sign of individuals' health and places greater emphasis on the dangers of extremely low weights.[31]

In consideration of these international and intranational differences, WHO released a study in 1998 arguing that individuals who are between a 25 and a 29 on the BMI should be categorized as overweight, whereas those at a 30 or above should be categorized as obese. Shortly after the WHO report, the U.S. National Institutes of Health adopted the lower threshold for categorizing individuals as overweight or obese, as did other health agencies. This had the result of putting twenty-five million more Americans into the overweight category, even though they did not gain an ounce.[32] Similar category adjustments led to the obesity rate in Hong Kong almost doubling from 30 percent 50 percent overnight.[33] I am less concerned with the validity of these particular adjustments and more concerned with their impact on bringing millions of people under the purview of health experts and categorizing millions of additional people as being in need of bodily change.

Regardless of what these data may actually indicate about changes to our collective sizes and health statuses, these examples reveal WHO as a major influence on the construction and framing of the obesity epidemic, the creation of large populations for monitoring, and ultimately the shaping of norms guiding individual attitudes and behaviors. In other words, these notions of obesity as a global *epidemic* standardize not only "classification, causality, responsibility, degeneracy," but also the "imaginable and pragmatic logics of cure" across incredibly large and diverse groups of people.[34] For example, following the WHO standardizations for children's growth specifically, one hundred four countries adopted WHO's weight-for-age metrics and thirty-six countries introduced new BMI-for-age classifications and monitoring.[35] These globalized metrics for bodily norms again position weight as a signifier of overall health. They also position weight reduction as inextricably linked to becoming healthier and avoiding "obesity-related diseases," which influences the way we may conceptualize our own bodies as well as national or governmental actions and policies to manage the bodies of citizenries.

These increasingly standardized understandings of fatness as a globesity epidemic give credence to Christine Halse's claim that WHO acts as a kind of modern panopticon due to its maintenance of disciplinary regimes in the name of public health.[36] WHO is thought to disperse management over the "problem of living" across nation-states and cities through the development of "complex apparatuses" that promote various "techniques of advice and guidance, medics, clinics, guides, and counselors."[37] Similarly, Kirsten Ostherr argues that WHO brings "local populations into global systems of knowledge" while legitimizing "the importance of bodily surveillance and control."[38] Furthermore, Emma Rich and John Evans claim that these examples of information gathering and measuring control broad populations (at a distance) while creating interventions and regulations that directly discipline individuals.[39] These conceptualizations of WHO parallel understandings of television, especially reality television, as a disciplinary apparatus by which forms of knowledge about health, fatness, and weight loss are disseminated to large populations around the world while participants on TV are surveilled and disciplined into specific bodily comportment. The information gathering and practices of entities like WHO provide content for television creators and foster a sense of significance and seriousness. But while television helps disperse disciplinary and bodily logics to audiences around the world, it also intrinsically resists those logics through various representational and narrative choices.

As discourses of the globesity epidemic sediment into a kind of "common sense," unfortunately so does fat stigmatization. Certain attitudes about fatness increasingly transcend national boundaries, particularly the notions that obesity is a health problem, fatness is socially undesirable, and weight gain and weight loss are tied to *personal responsibility*.[40] While these findings exist on a continuum with some nations and regions being more or less fat accepting than others, researchers ultimately argue that these distinctions seem to be blurring and that negative attitudes toward fatness seem to be spreading.[41] A writer for the *Calgary Herald* reports on this phenomenon: "Many countries that once associated curvy bodies with youth, fertility, wealth, and beauty have gobbled up North American's anti-fat prejudices and now associate obesity with laziness, lack of self-control, and moral failure."[42] Furthermore, *The Biggest Loser* itself may be helping to export or spread fat stigma. One study finds that watchers of the show are more likely to view fat individuals in negative ways because of the show's overt focus on personal responsibility—individual causes of and solutions to obesity—at the expense of exploring potential biological, social, environmental, industrial, or even just statistical factors in weight gain.[43]

Of course localities and nations are not homogenous, so this chapter is not about making general claims about large groups of people or about what one nation tolerates or does not tolerate as a whole; rather it's about the assumptions television producers make about locations and audiences.[44] In other words, it's about the industry lore that plays a role in how much or how little a television format like *The Biggest Loser* is translated from the original U.S. version to be exhibited across different international television markets. Switching out TV hosts and changing participants' weigh-in apparel may be important ways in which these shows are localized. Although they do not meaningfully alter the premise that weight loss is desirable or necessary, they may illuminate subtle differences in the levels of bodily shame or discipline, or punishing practices and extreme transformations, accepted by different countries and regions. In this chapter I argue that pro–weight loss, anti-fat attitudes are indeed present across all of these versions of *The Biggest Loser*; however, many international versions reject or minimize the most disciplining and shaming elements of the U.S. version. Television producers do this based on their own understandings of both the global saliency of weight-loss discourses (and popularity of makeover lifestyle television) and the norms of localized cultures or assumptions about localized audiences.

The international spread of *The Biggest Loser* as a format contradictorily reflects the resonance of globesity epidemic discourses and resistance to the extreme ways they are taken up by U.S. television. Internationally circulated television formats are thus useful for understanding tensions between globalized understandings of fatness, such as those constructed by WHO and other international NGOs, with local cultures, attitudes, and assumptions. Localizing content is the process of obscuring the global nature of television industries and media content, although both "localizing" *and* "universalizing" are always simultaneously present.[45] Albert Moran uses the pie metaphor to demonstrate how the globally standardized structure or blueprint of the television format acts as the pie crust while the pie filling reflects local influences and adaptations.[46] Sticking with food, Silvio Waisbord establishes through his "McTV" analogy that while global economics shape format circulation practices, local and national cultural influences generally shape content.[47] While these metaphors and analogies are useful for understanding the way a majority of formatting works, and the strategies behind formatting translation or adaptation, what is considered global *or* local seems increasingly blurred in regard to television programming of the globesity epidemic. Although I am not arguing that there exists a unified global culture, dominant discourses of the globesity epidemic are widely circulated, demonstrating broad acceptance of the premise that fat is something that individuals need to change. *The Biggest Loser* format represents one way in which television producers and channels endeavor to "overcome differences of national identity by emphasizing other markers of identity, such as . . . lifestyle interests." Since fatness is regularly framed as a health choice, as part of our lifestyles, it is viewed as transcending national identity. TV helps globesity discourses spread around the world, while globesity discourses help weight-loss TV spread around the world, too.

Televising Globesity

Reality makeover programs in general circulate well internationally.[48] Judging by the sheer number of documentaries and television series with content about weight loss and the obesity epidemic specifically, they seem to circulate quite well internationally too. Televised documentaries like *Weight of the Nation* (United States, 2012), *Weight of the World* (Canada, 2009), *Globesity: Fat's New Frontier* (Australia, 2012), *Muito Além do Peso* (*Way Beyond Weight*, Brazil, 2013), and *The Obesity Clinic* (Ireland, 2012), among others, all explore the context of the "globesity epidemic." National Geographic's *Half Ton World* (2013) travels internationally to document the ways in which individuals are, according to the show's narrator, "fighting for their livelihoods, freedoms, and even their lives." The show follows individuals in Mexico, India, and the United States in order to detail everyday experiences of fatness and document broad population changes, specifically Mexico being influenced by U.S. food exports and the impact of economic prosperity on India's growing middle class. Most of these programs directly reference WHO statistics, and all of them use BMI as a proxy for health status while framing weight loss as the route to improving overall health.

In addition to these made-for-TV documentaries, numerous TV series detail the everyday lives of fat individuals on their journeys to lose weight. Beyond *The Biggest Loser*, the United States is also home to Bravo's *Thintervention* (2010), VH1's *Celebrity Fit Club* (2005–), and Oxygen's *Dance Your Ass Off* (2009–2010) and *My Big Fat Revenge* (2013–). But the United States is of course not alone in producing programs specifically detailing and encouraging individual weight-loss narratives or weight-loss competitions. The United Kingdom has *Obese: A Year to Save My Life USA* (2012), *Fat: The Fight of My Life* (2013), *The Fat Fighters* (2012–2013), *Lorraine Kelly's Big Fat Challenge* (2010), *You Are What You Eat* (2004–2007), and *Supersize vs. Superskinny*. Likewise, Australia's Channel 9 developed *Big: Extreme Makeover* (2011), which follows individuals as they lose weight in order to "save their lives," "reinvent themselves," and "regain their former selves," as well as *Excess Baggage* (2012), which pairs Australian citizens and celebrities into teams competing to lose weight for money. Similarly, Canada has *Bulging Brides* (2008–2010) as well as *The Last Ten Pounds Bootcamp* (2007–2012). Also, Canada's Life Network program *Taking It Off* (2002) portrays five Calgarians in a competition to lose more weight than five citizen-dieters in Halifax. As part of a multiplatform initiative to help Canadians lose weight, called "Canada Weighs-In," the Canadian Broadcasting Company began airing *Village on a Diet* (2011), which follows the weight loss of a small British Columbia town with an obesity rate of 60 percent.

There is also Brazil's *Medida Certa* (*One Measure*, 2012), Germany's *The Big Diet* (2001–2002), and New Zealand's *Downsize Me!* (2005–2007), all of which focus on and track individuals as they lose or attempt to lose weight. Not only are there numerous iterations of weight-loss programs, as all of these examples attest, many of them also circulate internationally. For instance, Canada's *X-Weighted*, which was commissioned and is broadcast by the Canadian lifestyle channel Slice, is also shown on Sky UK, Turner Latin America, Foxtel, SBS (Belgium and Netherlands), TVNZ (New Zealand), TV4 (Sweden), Évasion (France), TV2 (Hungary), and TV5 (Finland). In addition to airing in the United States on MTV, *I Used to Be Fat* is also exhibited in the United Kingdom, Germany, Austria, Belgium, and the Netherlands, among other countries, on VIVA (a channel owned by MTV) and across MTV Latin America feeds covering Mexico, Colombia, Costa Rica, Chile, and Argentina. Weight-loss television texts also circulate widely on the internet as exemplified by the availability of full episodes of *Supersize vs. Superskinny*, *Obese: A Year to Save My Life*, and *Big: Extreme Makeover* on YouTube and other streaming services.

The Biggest Loser is perhaps the longest running and most widely circulated example of television directly addressing the globesity epidemic. The show debuted in the United States in 2004 with twelve individuals (out of the tens of thousands of individuals who go to casting calls or apply by submitting videos each season) competing to lose the largest percentage of body weight. The prize? A quarter of a million U.S. dollars. Each season begins the same way, with participants detailing why they consider themselves to be fat and the ways in which they believe fatness impedes their careers, interpersonal relationships, goal achievements, or self-esteem. Then contestants are put through either a bootcamp-style first workout or some other strenuous physical task that "proves" to participants how far they have "let themselves go." This frequently involves people passing out, vomiting, crying, and likely questioning why they signed up to participate on the show in the first place. Each subsequent episode's structure is the same: a rewards challenge, initial workout, last chance workout, last chance challenge, weigh-in, elimination challenge, and elimination vote. Although each episode follows a specific formula, individual weight-loss journeys become increasingly complicated as participants experience both weight-loss plateaus and weight gains, workout fatigue and injury, or a returning of previous "bad habits," all of which undermine the idea that transformation and learning and maintaining steadfast self-discipline to particular dieting and exercise regimens are straightforward even under "expert" supervision in a highly controlled and isolated environment. By season's end, the remaining contestants step on a giant scale-like apparatus—complete with flashing lights and sounds that change with the numbers of the scale increasing and decreasing in suspense—to reveal winners who typically lose between 40 and 60 percent of their original body weights. For season 9 winner, Michael Ventrella, this means losing 264 pounds. For season 15 winner, Rachel Frederickson, this means losing 155 pounds.

Despite debuting to critical disdain (a review in the *New York Times* refers to it as "obnoxious," while *Entertainment Weekly* calls it "mean-spirited," "manipulative," and "cruel"),[49] the show proved successful enough to inspire versions in the Netherlands (*De Afvallers*, or *The Slimmers*) and Brazil (*O Grande Perdedor*) in 2005, and versions in Argentina (*Cuestión De Peso*, or *Matter of Weight*), Australia, Finland (*Suurin Pudottaja*), Israel (*Laredet Begadol*, or *Going Down Big Time*), and Slovakia (*Super Body*) in 2006. As different international versions of the show popped up over the years while others fizzled out, *The Biggest Loser* transformed itself from a TV show into a global lifestyle brand, capitalizing on the increasingly global interest in "the perfectibility of the self."[50] *The Biggest Loser* has dozens of products including workout videos, such as *The Biggest Loser Cardio Max* and *The Biggest Loser At-Home Workout*, and *Biggest Loser*–themed weight-loss ranches in the United States, Germany, and Brunei. The show also developed lucrative integrated marketing arrangements with companies like Brita and Jennie-O, while running the Challenge America campaign, which encouraged Americans to "cut the junk" and "eat right on a budget" with the help of General Mills and Subway. Planet Fitness even started offering participants of Challenge America lower monthly gym rates.[51] These products and corporate partnerships helped market the show while the series itself worked to drive book and DVD sales, online enrollment in *The Biggest Loser* Club, and various licensed products.[52]

Each part of *The Biggest Loser* global lifestyle brand, including national or regional television formats, reflects globally dominant discourses of obesity that link large body size to poor health regardless of actual health status, position fatness as a necessary and legitimate reason for intervention, and frame fatness as the result of one's individual choices. Each version of *The Biggest Loser* espouses similar WHO statistics emphasizing how dire the obesity epidemic has become, with the organization saying that almost three million people around the world die each year as a result of being overweight or obese.[53] *The Biggest Loser's* own Dr. Huizenga offers another alarming (albeit uncited) statistic similar to the WHO's: "Worst case estimates put obesity as killing twenty-five thousand Americans a month." He then links this statistic to a commendation of *The Biggest Loser* for intervening and trying to "solve" the obesity epidemic: "We are seeing incredible results that we heretofore thought impossible. And as far as I'm concerned, Nobel Peace Prize here we come. We have a solution to a deadly disease. We try to use what we've learned here to help everyone in this country, everyone around the world. And to think that this is part of reality TV, which people sneer [at] and look down upon." As this statement exemplifies, and as discussed in chapter 3, *The Biggest Loser* sees itself as helping people on the show and as inspiring and empowering millions to take charge of their own health.[54] These kinds of self-congratulatory statements exist despite, or perhaps because of, the show being regularly criticized for talking about the importance of health while televising extreme and unhealthy weight-loss practices, or "quick and simplistic solutions to the complex problems of the self."[55]

With any adaptation or translation of television formats, producers work to make shows more appealing to local audiences according to their perceptions of what local (and sometimes regional) audiences will be receptive to. For example, Caroline Rhea, a U.S. comedian and actress, first hosted the U.S. version of *The Biggest Loser*, followed by Alison Sweeney, a popular daytime soap actress, while Sunil Shetty, a well-known Bollywood actor, hosted India's version, *Biggest Loser Jeetega*. These seemingly superficial changes make the show more recognizable and connected to different locales per media industry lore. These changes to different formats of *The Biggest Loser*, according to Tania Lewis, speak to a "complex process of articulation with local television traditions and with local cultures and lifestyles."[56] Sometimes this means very little translation, at least at first. For example, *The Biggest Loser U.K.* (2005–2006, 2009–2012) is most similar to the U.S. version, as it is similarly over-the-top in its first two seasons (or "series"), exhibited on cable channel Sky Living. The show's trainers, Angie Dowds and Mark Bailey, analogously motivate contestants through yelling, put them through the same kinds of elaborate physical challenges, and weigh them on large, light-filled scale apparatuses. However, after receiving less than stellar ratings, the show switched not only to another channel, ITV, but also to daytime, a more stripped-down daily format, and, according to the producers, a more compassionate tone.[57] Other times this means more significant translation for audiences who may not be as receptive to the extreme, dramatic, and overtly disciplinary solutions characteristic of the show.

In fact, *The Biggest Loser* (2006–2017) in Australia provides a useful case for understanding how the show is adapted for different international markets based on industry lore or cultural and audience assumptions. The Australian show's less confessional and less aggressively individualistic cultural norms in comparison to its U.S. counterpart can be seen throughout Australian makeover shows, which are less concerned with humiliation and competition and more concerned with creating a familiar, "neighborly" address. The show emphasizes transformation for the good of families and communities rather than individual entrepreneurialism.[58] In order to make *The Biggest Loser* work in Australia, FremantleMedia substantially reworked the format, making it nightly instead of weekly and creating a narrative that is more story driven, more "soap opera like."[59] A. J. Rochester, the host of *The Biggest Loser Australia*, explains that bodily transformations on its version are more realistic than those on the U.S. version: "In the American finale the curtains open and most of them walk through looking pretty damn good. You almost put them on a pedestal and go, 'Oh that's too hard' whereas in the Australian one there'll be different people at different points in their journey and that's more real. It's not driven by the perfect ending, because the perfect ending is that real people take time to change."[60] Although the first season of the Australian version did feature both U.S. trainers, Bob Harper and Jillian Michaels, which helped with brand recognition, not all viewers approved of their presence. One viewer lamented Australian participants being "bullied by obnoxious Americans," and readers voted it the "most stupid show" on Australian television.[61] Also like the U.S. version, non-show trainers and other fitness experts criticized the series for "promoting extreme and unhealthy methods" while "humiliating contestants."[62] Yet *The Biggest Loser Australia* became one of Australia's top rated shows in 2006,[63] with 1.3 million people tuning in each night.[64]

Later seasons featured Australian-based trainers who adopted less shaming styles of coaching compared to their U.S. counterparts. By 2010, it started distancing itself even more from the original U.S. format. According to one of the show's spokespeople, "Gone are the mind games of previous series. Instead it will be a more collaborative, educational and supportive environment."[65] While these tweaks to the format proved successful for a few years, lingering criticism of the show's practices and gradually dwindling ratings inspired *even more* changes to the format. By the spring of 2017 it shifted even further away from the drama and yelling-filled U.S. version of *The Biggest Loser* to become *The Biggest Loser: Transformation*.

The U.S. version purposely selects individuals believed to be "excessive,"[66] and continually makes it a point to always include "the biggest contestant ever!" with many participants desiring to lose, or are told by trainers and other experts on the show that they need to lose, one to two hundred pounds or more. However, *The Biggest Loser: Transformation* decided to start featuring individuals deemed more reflective of the bodies of viewers at home. The program touted itself as even less shaming, less extreme, and more relatable, practical, inspiring, useful, and kind.[67] The show also began focusing less on the numbers on the scale—typically the be-all and end-all on *The Biggest Loser*—to instead offer contestants the "whole package." For instance, this meant that therapy segments replaced "temptation challenge" segments, which were criticized for encouraging participants to consume thousands of calories of food.[68] The show's executive producer, Paul Leadon, explains that these changes are about updating the show to reflect evolving knowledge about nutrition and health science over the years since *The Biggest Loser* was first developed (as if the format was ever based on sound medical or scientific knowledge). Leadon also wanted to shed the show's image of "trainers yelling at people," calling it "just plain wrong" and more about "making moments for television" than weight loss.[69] These statements simultaneously reject the most overtly disciplining aspects of the show while maintaining its premise in accordance with dominant discourses of the obesity epidemic, offering an important example of the way television negotiates globesity discourses and its own role in disciplining at a distance.

Other international variations of the show include changing the name from *The Biggest Loser* to ones that sound more neutral. For example, the Russian version avoids the double entendre of "loser," instead going by *The Weighted People* (2015–), while the Ukrainian version opts for the happier sounding title *Weighted and Happy* (2011–). The Middle East's version of *The Biggest Loser* is also known by a more positive-sounding name: *The Biggest Winner (Ar-Rabeh Al-Akabar)*. According to Abdelfatah El-Masry, the programming director at the Middle East Broadcasting Center, or MBC (the first and perhaps largest private broadcaster in the Arab world), this change occurred to "keep it positive, not to add a negative twist." El-Masry elaborates, "In the Arab world they perceive these things somewhat different. . . . I think the programs that we've been creating or that we're doing now, they're more or less *feel-good* type of shows."[70] This format lasted four seasons between 2006 and 2009 on MBC, featuring participants from fourteen different countries, including Syria, Egypt, United Arab Emirates, Saudi Arabia, and Iraq, and filming in Lebanon. Several changes were made to the format, including fully clothed weekly weigh-ins (with some women wearing hijabs) instead of the flesh-revealing weigh-ins characteristic of the U.S. and U.K. versions, which reflects stricter norms of dressing and bodily display. This means that one of the most shame-inducing aspects of the show is removed; participants are not objectified to the same extent by the camera panning across participants' nearly nude bodies. Additionally, as Nourah Almaiman points out, contestants may carry each other in competition segments on the U.S. version, but there is no physical contact between contestants on *The Biggest Winner* in accordance with regional and religious norms.[71] The production company behind the show, IPROD, addresses these differences between formats in a statement: "As in the original production, the show gathered overweight men and women from all over the Arab world and challenged them to lose weight through a healthy diet and exercise. Highly attuned to Arab and Muslim cultural sensitivities about mixing the sexes, self-image, and public body display, IPROD led the adaptation of the original format, which included adding 55 daily episodes per season."[72]

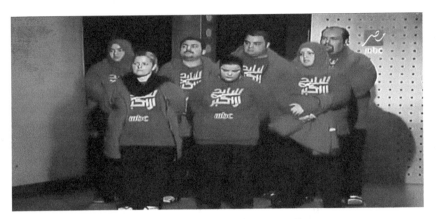

Figure 7   Contestants on *The Biggest Winner*

Thus, in addition to changes to weigh-ins and physical challenges, the daily format also reduces the potential televisual impact of the transformation of each episode, with less dramatic bodily changes achievable one day to the next compared to what can be achieved from week to week.

There are other subtle differences between the U.S. and Arab versions. For example, *The Biggest Winner* spends less time showing contestants talking about what they hate about themselves. Countries of origin are emphasized more in the Arab version compared to emphases on age and occupation in the U.S. version. Instead of representing success through pounds lost, on *The Biggest Winner* each pound represents a point *gained* (visualized with a plus sign instead of a minus sign).[73] Despite these seemingly subtle yet important differences, the main goal remains the same across each show: to lose the largest percentage of weight.

Another regional version of the show, *The Biggest Loser Asia* (2009–2010), features participants from Singapore, the Philippines, Thailand, Indonesia, Malaysia, and Hong Kong. The show debuted in the region on the Hallmark Channel after a year of exhibiting the U.S. version of *The Biggest Loser*, purportedly "priming the audience" and creating brand familiarity. Discussing the ways in which U.S. television generally needs to be translated for Asian audiences, Riaz Mehta, an executive producer on *The Biggest Loser Asia* and president of its production company, Imagine OmniMedia, explains, "People will always prefer local content because it is more relevant. But it has to be produced well. American shows are very American and the audience and appeal are limited."[74] In another interview he elaborates, "American shows are entertaining but Asians can't 'see' themselves in the show, therefore their level of engagement is lower than for a show made for Asia."[75] David Searl, a senior vice president of content partnerships for Star TV, echoes this sentiment to explain the logics behind translations of U.S. television for Asian audiences: "In America, the shows are often about the losers, about cutting people down, but that doesn't suit an Asian sensibility," adding that the success of *The Amazing Race Asia* was successful in Asia because it adopted a different tone from the U.S. version: "The show isn't about negativity, it's about teamwork, which resonates well in Asia."[76] But it appears that Asian audiences do not mind negativity if it's on a directly imported American show, considering that Searl adds, "Shows like *American Idol* are popular in Asia because Asians like to watch Americans being aggressive, but they generally don't like watching fellow Asians being aggressive."[77]

Upon its debut, *The Biggest Loser Asia* generated high enough ratings to make the Hallmark Channel the top channel in both Malaysia and Singapore during the show's timeslot (the channel was renamed Diva during the show's second season).[78] Similar to other iterations of the format, participants on *The Biggest Loser Asia* detail the individual "causes" of their fatness (eating fried chicken, rojak, satay, and chocolate while "being lazy") and individual "solutions" to their fatness (discipline, determination, and perseverance). One participant, Ayutthaya Allianz, alludes to cultural reasons behind his weight gain, saying that he's fat because "most Chinese seem to love fat people." He continues, "They think that being fat is good as it's a sign of wealth. My Chinese grandmother encouraged me to fatten up ever since I was a small."[79] Yet other participants discuss the ways in which they're discriminated against in the job market or feel interpersonally judged by others because of their fatness. Although participants on both *The Biggest Loser* and *The Biggest Loser Asia* cite experiences of fat stigma and discrimination, fewer individuals were eager to lose weight on TV in Asian countries compared to the United States. According to Searl, "Casting is also harder in Asia. Asians are less eager to open up," and they are not as "shameless" about "making fools of themselves."[80]

Like the U.S. version, *The Biggest Loser Asia* positions itself as performing an important public service for both the participants on the show and audiences at home. Karen Johnston, the programming director for NBC Universal Global Networks, contends that the show is about motivating viewers to "truly live life."[81] Mehta expands on this point, saying, "We wanted to do this because unlike most reality shows, this one is not purely entertainment-based. *The Biggest Loser* is about changing people's lives and not just the contestants on the show but also the millions of people watching at home. You don't have to be 80kg overweight to adopt the philosophies of the show."[82]

One of the trainers of *The Biggest Loser Asia*, Kristy Curtis, expresses the same notion: "Losing weight for them is not all about vanity, it is a means to change their lives and improve on what they have. . . . I hope to not just be able to coach the contenders towards a healthier lifestyle but inspire viewers as well. Finding out what lifestyle factors are affecting one's health is the key to achieving balance. . . . While there are some things in life you cannot control, you can take ownership and responsibility of your health through eating good food, thinking positively and keeping your body moving."[83] A season 1 participant, Zenny

Salihuddin, similarly abides by these public relations framings of the show, saying to participants auditioning for season 2 that *The Biggest Loser Asia* is not about quickly losing weight but about becoming healthier and happier, adding, "A contestant's major opponent is not the other contestants, but his or her weight."[84]

Also like the U.S. version of *The Biggest Loser*, *The Biggest Loser Asia* was met with resistance from off-show physical trainers and fitness experts. For example, the *Straits Times* in Singapore interviewed several medical doctors and fitness trainers who all argue that the "super-quick slim-downs" on reality TV should be given a "big fat 'no'" because losing weight too quickly can lead to health complications.[85] Similarly, Noel Chelliah, a trainer and blogger at the *Daily Muscle*, criticized the show for the high number of injuries among participants and wondered if it was because of a lack of proper pre-show health screening or inappropriateness of the exercises.[86] Chelliah also criticized the show for doing the exact opposite of Mehta's claims about the show focusing on health rather than drama and entertainment. The second season, in particular, does place a considerable emphasis on the tension between teams (with more scenes taking place in their living quarters to capture team infiltration and strategizing, all of which make for great television). Chelliah also faults *The Biggest Loser Asia* for spending less time portraying exercise segments compared to the U.S. version: "All I see are injuries, pain, a lack of emphasis on what the contestants are doing to actually lose that weight, and a strong focus on all the petty issues and drama that goes on."[87]

Beyond media industry lore, audience assumptions, and critical push-back, there are other important considerations in adapting U.S. television for other audiences: regulation. Searl argues that exhibiting a Western format without changing it "can be a minefield for Asian sensibilities," making shows "doomed to failure." Searl uses Thailand's production of *The Weakest Link* as an example of what can happen if international formats are not properly adapted for different local or national contexts. He explains that the show's "bitchy," "nasty" host "was so controversial that then Prime Minister Thaksin threatened in Parliament to take away the TV station's broadcast license because the show was offensive to Thai culture."[88] Similar debates occurred in Malaysia thanks to a huge influx of reality television programming along with *The Biggest Loser Asia*, such as *The Apprentice*, *Survivor*, and *The Amazing Race*. The deputy prime minister expressed concern that these shows "borrowed extensively from Western culture" and "could have a negative impact on viewers because some of the action wandered from the norms of local culture."[89] The deputy culture, arts, and heritage minister of Malaysia explained that the government would be evaluating reality television content, saying, "It is undeniable that some reality shows are probably unsuitable for Malaysian culture, tradition, customs, and religion, and can influence and poison the minds of youths."[90] One analysis of *The Biggest Loser Asia* points out that the stomach-baring sports bras characteristic of both the U.S. and Asian adaptations of *The Biggest Loser* are possibly against the Malaysia's Code of Ethics for Radio and TV.[91] These regulatory or governmental debates about content demonstrate another layer of assumptions about audiences—what they may deem suitable or unsuitable—that can influence the kinds of changes that are made in international adaptions of programming.

Whereas versions of *The Biggest Loser* in the United States, the United Kingdom, and Australia already assume audiences view fatness as a type of embodiment in need of transformation, the same was not necessarily true of the Philippines and its version, *The Biggest Loser Pinoy* (2011–2014). This iteration works to balance local understandings of fatness with standardized constructions of the globesity epidemic as a major health problem. Traditionally, "female" bodies were generally "preferred" (by women themselves and assumedly their romantic partners) throughout Southeast Asia and Pacific island nations.[92] In Filipino culture specifically, fat was more often associated with being healthy or eating properly.[93] However, WHO classifies three out of ten Filipinos as overweight or obese, with that number increasing every year and drawing a considerable amount of global attention to obesity rates across the region.[94] In an interview prior to *The Biggest Loser Pinoy*'s debut, host Sharon Cuneta explains that the show's goal is to teach Filipinos both at home and on the show how to lead healthier lives in order to build a stronger nation. Before the show's debut, the channel ABS-CBN aired a primer, *Bignating Pinoy* (2011), to introduce the topic and "to prove that obesity is a serious problem in the country" and that it "should be addressed."[95] One of the show's personal trainers, Chinggay Andrada, expressed a similar sentiment: "It's like a wake up call for a lot of people. And it's a problem or an issue that needs to be addressed as early as now here in the Philippines."[96]

Further demonstrating national and cultural differences in the way fatness is understood, the U.S. version of *The Biggest Loser* also addresses fatness in Southeast Asia and the Pacific islands. For example, Felipe and Sione, two Tongan cousins in the seventh season (2009) of *The Biggest Loser*, discuss the high rates of fatness on the Pacific island as being a result of the fat-accepting attitudes characteristic of Tongan culture (with some estimates categorizing 90 percent of Tongans as overweight or obese).[97] Felipe and Sione explain during their introductions on the first episode of the season, "Our parents are from the island of Tonga in the South Pacific and weight is a big thing to us. It becomes a part of the culture where it's normal to be big. In fact, if you're skinny, you're kind of frowned up. . . . We're trying to change the mentality of the Polynesian people that it's not okay to be big." After the show, as documented on the season 8 "Where Are They Now?" (2009) episode, the cousins start a Tongan fitness class and host a luau featuring "healthy" foods. In their words, they are celebrating salad instead of just using it as decorative garnish. Felipe says, "We're not going to be able to change tradition, but we can help tradition get better." In another step toward "helping" Tongan tradition, the 2010 *Biggest Loser* Thanksgiving special documents Sione traveling to Tonga for a meeting with the nation's princess to discuss spreading awareness about the problem of obesity and developing strategies for making the country "healthier" through weight loss.

Through both this example and *The Biggest Loser Pinoy*, I am not arguing that global influences necessarily "threaten" the integrity or autonomy of a kind of national identity or cultural differences but rather emphasizing that national identity can never "be isolated from the global, transnational relations in which it takes shape."[98] Whereas citizens and audiences in Pinoy and Tonga may have to be persuaded, at least to a certain degree, to buy in to weight loss generally and *The Biggest Loser* specifically, audiences in the United States and elsewhere are already assumed to view fatness as something to be rejected and changed. This may also mean that differing bodily norms may influence the levels or styles of discipline and shame assumed to be tolerable to audiences by TV producers and distributors.

Another important site for interrogating the circulation of global obesity epidemic discourses is the non–*Biggest Loser* program *Slimpossible*, which airs on Citizen TV (Kenya's largest station). As previously discussed, Kenya is currently framed as experiencing a dual problem: malnourishment and obesity. Like those of *The Biggest Loser Pinoy*, the weight-loss messages of *Slimpossible* are exhibited in contradistinction to some of the localized cultural and social understandings of fatness. In Kenya, carrying "some extra weight" is seen as preferable by many, and according to Lina Njoroge, a nutritionist featured on *Slimpossible*, "Many people don't even want to lose weight, because they say they don't want to lose their hips. They don't want to lose their behind."[99] This conceptualization of fatness—as neutral if not beautiful, rather than a problem to be managed—actually made it difficult to get participants to sign up for the show when it first started casting (not unlike the difficulties experienced by *The Biggest Loser Asia*). Njoroge explains, "People never used to talk about weight. They are very shy and nobody [wanted to] go on national television and talk about the struggles" to lose weight.[100] Much like *The Biggest Loser Pinoy*, *Slimpossible* is viewed as serving as an "awakening" to the dangers of obesity, according to Kenya's minister of health, who says it gets only minimal attention in Kenya compared to infectious diseases.[101] This "awakening" appears to be working as nearly a thousand people auditioned for later seasons of the show.

Slimpossible airs live on Saturday nights for twelve weeks. Many episodes start with a group dance where audiences at home are expected to join in (the dance leader instructs viewers, "Get some water, get a towel, and join in if you can!"). Most of the episodes feature host Lilian Muli checking in with participants to find out how they are doing and what exercises participants are learning to enjoy, with a few scenes of participants working out in the gym during the week. However, none of the participants are wearing body microphones during

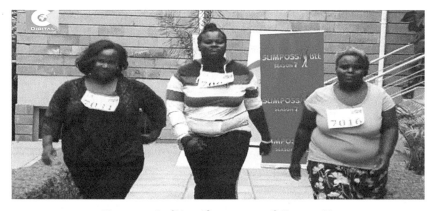

Figure 8   Auditions for season 7 of *Slimpossible*

workouts, like they do on most versions of *The Biggest Loser*, which means there are no trainers yelling in the faces of participants but just shots of people on exercise bikes with music playing in the background. The workouts themselves are much more ordinary and less intense (they're not dragging planes down runways or running marathons by the second week). When participants pause when running up the stairs, none of the trainers swoop in to yell at them drill-sergeant-style, but demonstrate understanding that sometimes people need to pause and catch their breath. A lot of the participants are shown working out at home, as none of them are quarantined on a weight-loss ranch like on *The Biggest Loser*. Instead they integrate physical activity and dietary changes into their everyday lives. Overall, per a reviewer of the show, "the show is not about rewarding contestants who lose the most weight, it's about getting Kenyans to rethink their headlong dive into convenience eating."[102]

Unlike *The Biggest Loser* in the United States, *Slimpossible* is all about moderation. Some of the participants lose twenty kilograms (or forty pounds) across the twelve weeks, which averages to a still substantial three pounds a week. There is not a specific *Slimpossible* diet; instead each participant has an individualized plan taking into account age, metabolism, and even dietary preferences. There are no banned foods or "bad" foods, per Njoroge, who explains, "On a healthy eating plan, you're not on punishment. If you have a treat, you know what to do after that." The show's nutritionist even uses the example of a participant eating a cookie as a positive aspect of weight loss (rather than an example of "cheating" or a slip in personal responsibility) because health is not about deprivation but instead about moderation, about finding balance. In fact, contestants are even cautioned against working out too much, not resting enough, and not eating enough. Njoroge explains, "If someone loses too much weight and they're not doing it right, it shows" through their triglyceride levels and other bodily metrics like cholesterol and blood sugar. The host then reminds participants, "You need to eat to burn!"

Slimpossible also emphasizes body positivity, making the show, according to Muli, a "transformation of confidence" rather than just a transformation of the body. While the show does frame fatness as unhealthy, it focuses less on individual blame to instead consider the environmental, social, genetic, and psychological aspects of one's life that may contribute to fatness. Carol, one of the experts on *Slimpossible*, says of the participants during the season 6 finale, "Blaming them or saying it's [fat] ugly . . . their fault . . . is really painful." Instead of shaming individuals pre–weight loss, *Slimpossible* celebrates each woman throughout the process. In a season 7 promotional commercial, the women auditioning for the show strut up and down the sidewalk as if they're in a fashion show. Each week, participants dress up for the live episode and are told by Muli how lovely they look ("From the way you're walking, you know you look hot!"). They enter onstage every Saturday night wearing the latest fashions and dancing to the applause of the live audience. Participants do not have to wait to lose weight before feeling good and being confident in themselves. Compounding the positivity, each episode features a chyron scrolling live tweets from viewers of the show, almost all of which are motivational and congratulatory, celebrating how hard the participants are working and how great they look (even if they have not lost a pound). The show thrives on positive reinforcement rather than the negative, disciplining reinforcement characteristic of *The Biggest Loser* in the United States. For instance, speaking at the season 6 finale, Liz, a contestant, says that whether they lost five kilos or twenty, the show celebrates the participants. In fact, many of the women look the same on the final episode as they did on the first, losing minimal to moderate amounts of weight per *The Biggest Loser*'s standards, but dramatic bodily reveals are unimportant to the show. What matters to *Slimpossible* is that individuals are, indeed, becoming healthier and happier, if not necessarily skinner.

Conclusion

As these seemingly subtle yet important differences between international weight-loss television series demonstrate, television balances the constructions of and assumptions about local cultures and audiences with global media industry lore and international health discourses. Tania Lewis reminds us, "The makeover format speaks neither solely to the 'national ordinary' nor to a purely universalizing televisual culture of Euro-American lifestyles and consumption, but rather to a television industry and culture marked by increasingly complex negotiations between globalizing forces and domestic concerns and contexts."[103] Yet we must also remember that makeover culture—in the form of weight-loss television—is "dialectical, marked by incessant border skirmishes over questions of elitism and populism, power and subordination, knowledge and exclusion, resistance and consent."[104] So while the global spread of *The Biggest Loser* demonstrates the normalization and standardization of discourses of fatness as globesity, fatness as a global health threat, looking at local format changes can elucidate challenges to televised disciplinary logics in the United States.

While international formats of *The Biggest Loser* make adjustments to the format based on industry lore and assumptions about audiences and local, national, or regional cultures, that does not mean that the U.S. version remains a static entity from which to replicate. In fact, *The Biggest Loser* "did an extreme makeover of its own" after the first season by focusing more on the "heartrending stories of participants whose transformations were tougher than they'd imagined."[105] The show became more "character-driven" and serious, downplaying games and accentuating personal stories. J. D. Roth explains that this is the key to *The Biggest Loser* becoming one of the most watched shows during the late aughts: "All of a sudden we were able to put some of the great human stories into the show. You could literally see the change in the ratings and the goodwill of the brand. And this is what the future of reality television hinges on—its ability to find real people that other real people will want to watch."[106] Although this change does not alter the underlying premise of the show, these emphases on stories create an important interplay between narrative tensions, participant identifications, and the disciplinary and surveillance logics advanced by the show. This interplay then exposes disciplinary discrepancies, inconsistencies, and the show's own illogicalities, undermining the dominant logics of the obesity epidemic and challenging TV's ability to govern at a distance, which is where we turn in chapter 5.

5   Exercising Control and the Illogics of Weight-Loss Television

"The gym was closed. It was a sign I wasn't meant to go to the gym," Sukhda explains on episode 3 of *Revenge Body with Khloe Kardashian* (2017–), adding, "I will literally Uber from my dorm to my school, which is less than a mile." Sukhda is a college student who says she was raised like a princess in New Deli, India, but struggled to adjust to the United States, where she moved for school. Sukhda tells Khloe and her new personal trainer provided by the show, La, that she orders pizza every night for dinner and that she considers walking to be "for poor people." From the beginning of the episode, it's clear that Sukhda is a unique participant who is either going to struggle or be one of the show's biggest transformations. Khloe emphasizes this point by saying, "I feel like this is going to be very difficult for you since you don't even like to walk, but this journey will probably be so rewarding for you."

At Sukhda's first workout with La, she arrives forty minutes late and complains, "Did you guys forget I don't walk?" La is not amused and questions Sukhda's commitment to the program and to her own transformation. The scene cuts to an interview segment with La saying to the camera, "She's really entitled and she thinks the world revolves around her," before Sukhda replies in her own interview segment, "She snapped at me and I wanted to throw her off the hill, but that's illegal in America." Despite the dramatic start to Sukhda's "transformation," she begrudgingly begins her workout. She slowly sinks into a slight squatting position, groaning, grimacing, and rolling her eyes with every movement. La struggles to get Sukhda to take the process seriously throughout the episode, while Sukhda seems to be taking pleasure in subverting the rules. In a phone-captured, confessional-style segment, Sukhda talks about eating ice cream "just because she can," makes cinnamon rolls, and later jokes to La that she drank half a bottle of tequila the night before a morning workout. Sukhda also refuses to send La photographic evidence that she's working out or taking yoga classes on her own (because she's not). By the six-week point, Sukhda has gained back five pounds from the small amount she lost since starting the show. This weight gain is enough for La to give up on Sukhda, saying, "Outside this gym, you're not doing what you're supposed to be doing. You're laughing and smiling, but it's really not funny. . . . At this point, I'm just going to have to let you go from this journey." Before leaving *Revenge Body*, Sukhda explains to producers that the show is a waste of time and that no one actually wants to transform; instead, they're on TV because they want to be famous.

While Sukhda is the first to be cut from the show before completing the twelve-week weight-loss transformation, she is not the last. By episode 6, Brittany is also asked to leave *Revenge Body*, but not before the show fully demonstrates her noncompliance. Brittany is exposed for drinking blended coffee containing a banned substance (dairy!), and producers confront her on the street when it's reported she's eating another banned substance (chips!). At one point, Khloe gives her an ultimatum, "Either buckle down and take it seriously, or say, 'You know what? I don't have the drive and dedication in me right now.'" But the confrontations and ultimatums irritate Brittany. She takes off her microphone, sets it on the sidewalk, and walks away. However, Brittany's journey on *Revenge Body* does not end there. She returns to her nutritionist (assumedly at the request of producers) to be further scolded for eating a filet-o-fish sandwich and for her body fat percentage going up from 30.5 percent to 33.55 while on the show. At this point, the nutritionist informs her that he will no longer work with her, and it's clear the producers asked her to attend the appointment just to end her storyline on their terms instead of hers.

Revenge Body positions itself as a makeover for individuals who have gained weight from past experiences of trauma or major life changes (usually romantic breakups), not unlike dozens of other weight-loss television series probing the personal experiences that "trigger" weight gain. The show frames itself as a more empowering and body-positive version of the reality makeover subgenre, downplaying numbers on the scale and emphasizing how participants feel emotionally and spiritually. The same combination of contradictory postfeminist discourses—of empowerment through consumption, microdermabrasion, tooth veneers, and waist trainers—is also found in Kardashian's book, *Strong Looks Better Naked* (2015) and the way she documents her own weight-loss experience and supportive glam team on her social media accounts and the family's show, *Keeping Up with the Kardashians* (2007–). Khloe explains during the opening credits, "Growing up, people called me the fat, funny sister . . . until I started working out, eating right, and putting myself first. Now I'm helping others transform because a great body is the best revenge!" And while some participants do feel "transformed" by episode's end, Sukhda and Brittany demonstrate, at least according to Khloe, that "not everything has a fairytale ending."

Khloe's program is one of the newest shows in a long line of weight-loss television programs emerging in the mid- to late 2000s corresponding with growing concern over the size of our bodies, including *The Biggest Loser, Extreme Weight Loss, Heavy, I Used to Be Fat, Thintervention* (2010), *Too Fat for 15* (2010–2011), *Diet Tribe* (2009), *Love Handles* (2011), *Dance Your Ass Off* (2009–2010), and *Shedding for the Wedding* (2011). To television creators and executives, weight-loss programs have a built-in audience of people who identify with bodily displeasure, or the experiences of both fatness and the social stigma surrounding fat bodies. Iterating this perception, Mark Koops, a co–executive producer on *The Biggest Loser*, says, "It is a very relatable subject matter and one that is only becoming more and more timely with the continued rise of obesity and the cost of obesity."[1] In fact, around the debut of NBC's *The Biggest Loser* in 2004 and at its peak in 2009, over ten million people tuned in each week (making it the most watched prime-time TV behind football games). However, with each subsequent year—and a growing number of controversies—its viewership shrunk to an average of three million viewers during its seventeenth season, inspiring rumors of its cancellation in the summer of 2017.[2] ABC's workout and diet-focused version of weight-loss television, *Extreme Weight Loss*, which documents a year in each participant's life over the course of each episode rather than the weekly group weigh-ins and eliminations on *The Biggest Loser*, debuted to seven million viewers in 2011, but it also dropped to just two million viewers per episode by its cancellation in 2015. Of course, the lowest rated episodes of *The Biggest Loser* and *Extreme Weight Loss* would be considered strong for the numerous weight-loss shows across cable channels, particularly MTV's *I Used to Be Fat*, A&E's *Heavy*, TLC's *Fat Chance*, and E!'s *Revenge Body with Khloe Kardashian*, which averages just a few hundred thousand viewers per episode.

Despite subtle differences in format and storytelling, these series all reflect dominant discourses of the obesity epidemic, namely that the size of our bodies is primarily a matter of how much we eat and how much we move, rather than just another state of being or a complex issue influenced by our environments, cultural traditions, industries, families, psychologies, and physiologies. As demonstrated in previous chapters, these fat-focused television shows typically position themselves as benefiting individuals, changing lives, and operating in a sense of the public interest, which downplays the increased scrutiny many of these shows are under for their extreme, and potentially dangerous, practices. According to J. D. Roth, a producer on both *The Biggest Loser* and *Extreme Weight Loss*, "For some of these people, this is their last chance . . . and in a country right now that is wrestling with health care issues and the billions of dollars that are spent on obesity issues per year, in a way what a public service to have a show that inspires people to be healthier."[3] Despite paying lip service to working in the public interest, *The Biggest Loser* and *Extreme Weight Loss* are ultimately about entertainment. And that entertainment, according to James Fell, a critic for the *Guardian*, comes at the cost of "shaming contestants, encouraging dangerous exercise regimens, promoting impossible weight-loss targets."[4] Adding to the criticism and pushing back against the notion that *The Biggest Loser* operates in the public interest, obesity physician Dr. Yoni Freedhoff complains that the show is "more powerful than any public health message," which is a problem because he also considers it to be "the most god-awful dangerous thing to happen to weight management in history. . . . *The Biggest Loser* is everything that's wrong with weight-loss in America."[5]

Television and Makeovers

Although reality makeovers proliferate TV today, makeover and transformational programming have a long history both on television and throughout American culture. Robert Thompson argues that transformation and reinvention are deeply embedded into the fabric of the United States, adding, "In a very real sort of way, the history of the United States is one big fat makeover show."[6] As early as the 1950s, daytime television programs like *Glamour Girl* (1953–1954) "celebrated the beautification of women" through before-and-after transformations.[7] Another show reinforcing narrow constructions of femininity on television via makeovers is *Queen for a Day* (1955–1964), which billed itself as the "Cinderella Show" by offering participants "glorious transformation via rampant consumerism."[8] In addition to these overt transformations, Tania Lewis reminds us that television's history is full of daytime cooking, home improvement, and talk shows that also emphasize self-improvement through the help of advisors and experts.[9] Contemporary television is, of course, now home to dozens of makeover series (thanks to the explosion of reality television throughout the 2000s) that typically reinforce the power and potential of transformation through consuming particular goods and disciplining individual thoughts and behaviors.[10]

Contemporary reality television is generally understood in relation to surveillance and discipline, and research on makeover programming in the neoliberal context provides an important theoretical foundation for making sense of weight-loss reality television. Laurie Ouellette and James Hay look specifically at makeover reality television and its use of hidden camera surveillance, public humiliation, and other controlling techniques.[11] They argue on-screen discipline works to prevent others, specifically television viewers, from misbehaving in the future. Reality television makeovers or interventions teach viewers at home how to be independent and self-disciplined as opposed to reliant on the state. According to Ouellette and Hay, "The political rationality of the life intervention is that people who are floundering can and must be taught to develop and maximize their capacities for normalcy, happiness, material stability, and success rather than rely on a public 'safety net.'"[12] The logics or rationalities of televised life interventions reinforcing messages of self-discipline, self-control, self-governance, self-help, and other emphases on the self then extend beyond programming, circulating throughout the late capitalist context and influencing everything from discussions of social welfare and pushes for privatizing traditionally public systems to constructions of the obesity epidemic. Numerous other studies look at the way reality television inspires change and transformation, from *What Not to Wear* (2003–2013) and *Makeover Story* (2000–) to *Extreme Makeover* (2002–2007) and *Queer Eye for the Straight Guy* (2003–2007), which all work to teach us that our appearances are never good enough and that change is imperative to becoming an "acceptable" individual.[13] *The Biggest Loser* is considered to operate in much the same way by working to shape our behaviors, educate subjects, discipline the "noncompliant," and generally help differentiate between "good" and "bad" citizens.[14] But just as *Revenge Body* attests, with its team of celebrity trainers, nutritionists moonlighting as psychotherapists, and "glam teams," transformation is neither constant nor easy. And sometimes transformation is not achieved at all.

This chapter troubles notions of television governing at a distance or operating as an extension or replacement of government despite the tendency to frame television in such a capacity. The programs discussed in this chapter are articulated most specifically to the communication and health policies as well as media industry discourses discussed in chapters 2 and 3. These programs are also articulated to dominant discourses of the fat body—hence their prominence in policy and industry discussions—which reinforce the notion that fatness is both a worldwide epidemic and a matter of individual choices and individual responsibilities. However, these programs are also rife with disciplinary discrepancies, inconsistencies, ineffectiveness, and even failure. Because they are ultimately supposed to be entertaining, attempts to discipline, surveil, and transform occur simultaneously with fostering participant (or character) identification, building dramatic tension, and creating suspenseful and engaging television narratives that are more likely to be enjoyed by viewers (and thus achieve higher ratings and increased advertising revenue). Weight-loss reality television in the makeover tradition, then, needs to be considered as *television*, as a type of content that can be disciplining or governing as well as entertaining and pleasurable (and, perhaps, both socially damaging and operating in a sense of the public interest, as discussed in chapter 2). This chapter examines episodes of *Extreme Weight Loss* and of *The Biggest Loser, I Used to Be Fat*, and *Heavy* to understand the ways in which television's multiple roles serve to reinforce dominant discourses of the obesity epidemic while implicitly resisting and complicating them through representations and narratives of fatness. While TV may work to discipline the body both on-screen and at home, TV also demonstrates the ways in which narratives and bodies may intrinsically resist—while participants on-screen may explicitly resist—the logics of televised transformation.

Explaining Fat Embodiment

We're introduced to Christy (season 4, episode 11) on *Extreme Weight Loss* as she opens her fridge for a snack. She is thirty-six years old and describes herself as two hundred twenty pounds over her ideal weight, explaining to the camera, "I've always been overweight. I was born a big baby." Yet Christy believes she gained excess weight because she grew up in an emotionally repressed family that never said "I love you" and endured bullying throughout elementary and high school. At one point, Christy tears up as she describes to the camera how she attempted to kill herself at a young age, saying, "I got it in my head one

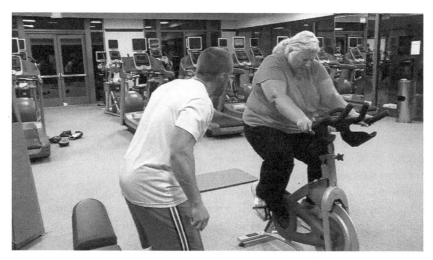

Figure 9   Christy's "fight or flight workout" on the "Kenny and Christy" episode of *Extreme Weight Loss* (2014)

morning that the only way to not get bullied anymore was to not live anymore. I couldn't do anything about being fat . . . the only thing I could do was end my life." This kind of emotional storytelling is typical of *Extreme Weight Loss*, which follows one or two participants under the guidance and surveillance of trainer Chris Powell and his wife and fellow trainer, Heidi Powell. Like Christy, Robert and Raymond, who are twins featured in the first episode of season 5, explain their weight gain as the result of their mother's incarceration, their father's abandonment, and the responsibility of raising their younger siblings at just thirteen years old. They say they turned to food for the comfort they did not receive from their parents, and by their mid-twenties both participants weighed over four hundred pounds.

Other traumatic events detailed on *Extreme Weight Loss* include the death of a loved one, divorce, illness, and even experiences of childhood abuse. On the first episode of the fourth season, Ty explains that he is fat for two reasons: "gorging on food" after baseball practices and using food to fill the void caused by his absentee alcoholic mother. In a later episode, another participant, Bruce (season 4, episode 4), gains weight after his father is sent to prison for sexually abusing both him and several of his football teammates. Another episode follows Melissa (season 4, episode 5), who gains one hundred fifty pounds following the suicide of her husband who suffered from posttraumatic stress disorder after his return from military service in Afghanistan. Sara (season 4, episode 10) says she gained weight trying to cope with being bullied because of her short stature caused by achondroplasia, and Alyssa (season 3, episode 9) believes she gained almost three hundred pounds while dealing with her mother's death following a car accident.

Although these examples represent the "bad lifestyle decisions" so often discussed in relation to the obesity epidemic, the events detailed through these stories frame these decisions as understandable. Shows like *Extreme Weight Loss* represent participants as victims of their circumstances, as sufferers or experiencers of undeniably traumatic life events that make coping a particularly arduous task, instead of just being framed as lazy. Even if these series still focus on the individual as opposed to broader social issues, cultural understandings, or the relationship between industries and policies, they do step away from the overtly shaming, and thus disciplining, aspects emphasized in other makeover or transformational television programming.[15] However, even though these shows may mitigate assertions that fatness is connected to laziness or indiscipline, they do reinforce it as being connected to experiences of trauma or emotional issues stemming from significant life events rather than a neutral state of being.

These personal stories, in addition to adding dramatic tension to the televised narratives, also humanize participants and potentially foster feelings of empathy or compassion among viewers. We learn from these stories that being smart, caring, lovable, and hardworking are not characteristics reserved for thin individuals. Instead of positioning participants as objects or as abject,[16] *Extreme Weight Loss, I Used to Be Fat, Heavy,* and, to a slightly lesser extent, *The Biggest Loser* humanize participants to create identification and emotional attachment for audiences, which downplays the shame and judgment encouraged elsewhere in the makeover TV landscape (even if inadvertently). Furthermore, these examples also complicate Gareth Palmer's assertion that reality shows about "large people" or "legitimate targets" (to use his terminology) frame the "failure to lose weight [as] symptomatic of a faulty self and nothing else."[17] Instead, the extended histories of individuals on these shows position the "faulty self" as not being a fault originating from the self. Through access to discussions between one participant on *Heavy,* Sharon (season 1, episode 3), and her therapist, it is revealed and reframed as *understandable* that Sharon gained over one hundred pounds after the death of her mother and the suicide of her son within a short period. As many of these narrative examples illustrate, the televisual components that reinforce messages of individualized fault or the need for self-discipline also simultaneously contradict or at least trouble those messages with more complex narratives and elaborate contextual details of each person's journey. Even the less dramatic reasons cited for weight gain on *I Used to Be Fat,* such as having an overprotective mother, divorced parents, or a large Italian family that expresses love through food, exemplify that fatness is more complex than a faulty self, or fault is at least partially attributable to external influences or actors outside of the self.

This attention to personal history is one of the primary ways in which weight-loss reality television programs differ from other series in the makeover tradition. June Deery notes that makeover programs usually offer only limited and depoliticized personal histories in an attempt to achieve broader viewer identification.[18] However, weight-loss TV typically spends a great deal of time at the beginning of each episode describing individual situations and discussing both past and present personal, familial, and social lives, and often returns to those stories throughout each episode. Greater attention to individual histories is perhaps possible because focusing on the body itself already achieves a kind of broad identification with audiences (*everyone* has a body). Plus, the categorization of two-thirds of individuals, at least in the United States, as having a BMI outside of the normatively constructed "healthy" range, along with a long history of representational homogeneity across media texts as well as advertising and marketing strategies that work to make people feel "less than," likely leads to these all-too-common feelings of individual discontent and desire for weight loss. Although viewers may not necessarily identify with the "bizarre" or "dated" wardrobes and styles featured on *Ambush Makeover* (2003–2005) or the cluttered living rooms appearing on *Clean House* (2003–), a wide range of viewers can unfortunately identify with feelings of discontent—and even outright hatred— toward the composition and appearance of their own bodies. Or at least they can identify with societal discourses framing fat bodies in such ways.

However, not every participant is granted the same level of televisual compassion, with participants on *The Biggest Loser* receiving the most personal blame, shame, and judgment from "experts" on the show. In addition to traumatic life events triggering weight gain, other "irresponsible life choices" are also highlighted. One of the ways in which these poor dietary choices are visually conveyed is through camera shots cataloging refrigerator, cupboard, and employee break room contents, or shots of participants consuming stereotypical "junk foods" or being sedentary while playing video games or watching television. For example, Bruce (season 4, episode 4) on *Extreme Weight Loss* is depicted drinking over one hundred ounces of Mountain Dew for breakfast. Also on *Extreme Weight Loss*, Ty (season 4, episode 1) is shown not only eating from a bucket of Kentucky Fried Chicken (the horror!) but also dumping loose pieces of fried batter into his mouth and washing it down with a liter of Coca-Cola. Depicting both inactivity and food consumption, Cassie (season 4, episode 9) is shown eating fast food and watching television while her husband watches a different television mounted on the opposing wall. Many participants are also shown eating fast food in their vehicles, including Christy (season 4, episode 11) going to McDonald's after a night of drinking and Tom, a season 1, episode 1 participant on *Heavy*, ordering six junior bacon cheeseburgers and three orders of spicy nuggets at Wendy's. All of these are examples of the "bad habits" participants must disavow according to "experts" across weight-loss programs, and they support the "necessity" or legitimacy of the televised weight-loss intervention.[19] Yet even these "bad habits" are sometimes framed as relatable, as an unfortunate part of what it means to live in the United States in the contemporary moment, when half of all individuals report eating fast food once a week,[20] when eating out is a way to socialize, celebrate, and experience pleasure,[21] and when relying on convenience foods is a way to manage stress and juggle family responsibilities.[22] Like Georgeanna (season 4, episode 8) says to the camera during her introduction on *Extreme Weight Loss*, "I got caught up in being a mom and forgot who Georgeanna is."[23]

These personal stories can also reinforce the notion that fatness is undesirable or a "before state" to be rejected, even if they trouble discourses of individual blame. Many of these stories are also told while participants stand in front of mirrors and examine their nude or near-nude bodies, and as Brenda Weber points out, these scenes are typical of makeover programs because they provide visual evidence of the necessity and desirability of the makeover. Weber elaborates, "These moments when the body's flaws are put on display cast makeover subjects as not only shameful, but grotesque; a conceit of degradation that similarly positions the makeover intervention as nothing short of miraculous."[24] Palmer similarly argues that the extreme close-ups depicting participants as "shameful" and also as submitting themselves for "treatment" are a ritualized part of reality TV transformations. Participants and viewers at home are also supposed to reject the body by facing the reading of it as a deformity and then committing to change.[25] Kathie (season 4, episode 2) on *Extreme Weight Loss* exemplifies this process well. While tearfully looking in the mirror, she lifts her stomach, sighs, and says, "I fed my pain." On season 4, episode 6 of *Extreme Weight Loss*, David also lifts his stomach while saying, "This is the reason I avoid going to places. I'm huge, sloppy. I'm an embarrassment to [my girlfriend]." Similarly, on episode 5 of *Heavy*, Flor holds her bare stomach as she says, "This is what it looks like when you allow food to take over your life." And Lindy, who appears on episode 4 of *Heavy*, pats her stomach as she cries, "This is my fat, fat, fat, fat, fat stomach. I really want this to go away. When I look in the mirror now, I just want to say 'What the fuck happened to you? How did you let this happen?'" This negative emotionalism, which Weber argues is reserved for describing the "before-state" of bodies,[26] is especially present when Charita, a season 4, episode 1 participant on *Extreme Weight Loss*, cannot even look in the mirror at her own body because she neither wants to see herself nor wants television viewers at home to see her. Instead, she begins crying and shuts the door on the camera crew attempting to film her. These moments work to produce shame, according to Weber, Palmer, and other scholars like Martin Roberts, but they also work to produce compassion, understanding, and empathy.[27] They work to make us care about and potentially identify with the participants on these shows. The pain expressed by participants as they discuss their perceived bodily flaws humanizes them in tension with the surveilling and objectifying camera that instead works toward producing feelings of revulsion, embarrassment, or shame. The transformations represented on these shows are not superficial; they're not our wardrobes or homes, they're our bodies. Bodies that we've collectively been led to believe are fundamental to who we are, and bodies that many fat people are led to believe are ugly, undesirable, and in need of change.

These "shame-inducing" scenes also function somewhat differently because they do not need to convince participants to desire change, as participants already want change. Weber discusses the way makeover programs involve friends and family who "out" individuals as needing makeovers. For example, on *What Not to Wear*, friends and family members spy on unsuspecting individuals to gather convincing evidence that an intervention and makeover are needed. On weight-loss programs, however, individuals sign themselves up. *Extreme Weight Loss* consistently emphasizes that participants on the show write letters to Powell asking for his help and then express joy and gratitude upon being "chosen" for the "transformation of their life." Over two hundred fifty thousand people applied to be on the U.S. version of *The Biggest Loser* in 2007 alone![28]

This difference between desiring an "intervention" and being convinced to consent is connected to another important difference across weight-loss series in comparison to other makeover shows: the source of "before-body" criticism. Makeover programs typically feature friends, family, strangers passing on the street, the program's "experts," or all of these groups together offering detailed and likely hurtful critiques of the participants to convince them of the need for a makeover. Weber argues that on makeover programs this destroys the "palliative that the ugly person is his or her own worst critic" and that his or her "internalized invective pales in comparison to what others think of them."[29] However, weight-loss programs tend to do the opposite. Instead of friends, family, or "experts" critiquing each participant's body, participants primarily critique their bodies themselves (of course what they say about their bodies is likely influenced by producer or "expert" questions and statements off camera). First, it would likely be read as cruel for others to critique the aesthetic of the *body* because it's an innate part of who we are rather than something we can take off or move in and out of. Second, when program "experts," such as medical doctors and trainers, do critique the body, it is always in terms of health, which is considered a more objective form of assessment than aesthetic critiques of the body.

However, these understandings of health itself are themselves combinations of aesthetic preferences and scientific projects rooted in cultural and moral understandings of fatness as problematic.[30] Although the appearance of fat may be reason enough to warrant a body intervention to some, health reasons are legitimized in the context of the obesity epidemic. This is not to say that some shows do not insult their participants' appearances or actions. In fact, the host of the United Kingdom's *Fat Families* (2010) refers to participants as "dumpy donuts," tells them to stop putting food into their "cake holes," and instructs people to get off their "wobbly bums." But even these examples are not directly critiquing the appearance of participant bodies, and the host's comments are "justified" because, as the host explains, he is a "former fatty."

Despite these subtle differences between weight-loss series and other reality shows, weigh-in scenes do work to produce shame consistent with other makeover programs. Participants on *I Used to Be Fat* weigh themselves in their own homes with their trainers and family members present. Similarly, participants on *Heavy* are weighed in privately (as private as can be with a camera crew present) either in a doctor's office or in the workout area once they arrive to the Hilton Head Island fitness resort. These kinds of weigh-ins are framed as necessary for participants learning the "severity" of their bodily situations; they may produce tears but are not overly dramatized like the ones on *The Biggest Loser*, meaning there is no giant scale-like apparatus with flashing lights and displays of numbers moving up and down to slowly zero in on the contestant's weight.

While makeover logics, according to Weber and Palmer, use these scenes to induce shame, they can also be read as excessive, unnecessary, or even cruel. Across the first three seasons of *Extreme Weight Loss*, participants are weighed in using a freight scale on the loading dock of the California Health and Longevity Institute. This practice occurs under the guise of the facility—specifically designed for health and weight loss, no less—not having a scale capable of handling the size of participants on the show. Despite using personal participant histories to generate audience attachment, the use of a loading dock freight scale positions fat individuals as beyond the size of human possibility and more like an object to be measured. Similarly, starting in the fourth season of *Extreme Weight Loss*, weigh-ins occur more often in public spaces. For instance, Charita is weighed in at a heavily populated outdoor mall in downtown Denver. Powell instructs her to remove her shirt and shoes and step on the scale. When Charita hesitates in front of the large crowd of strangers gathered around her, Powell urges, "This process is about not hiding anymore." In a similar vein, another of the show's participants, Brandi, is forced to weigh in on an auditorium stage following a beauty pageant. When Brandi hesitates after Powell also instructs her to take off her shirt and step on the scale in front of a large group of people, he reassures her, "It's all about letting go."

Regardless of the questionable, television-drama-enhancing justifications for the practice, the visual documentation of fat bodies in these types of scenes, according to Palmer, reinforces fat as signifying a "loss of control" or an "absence of will," while providing "license to increase surveillance and hypervigilance for well-being."[31] To Weber, makeover shows support messages of self-governance by this showcasing of bodies in "need" of self-discipline and by reproducing a critical social gaze that "exposes the shame of the 'ugly' body as it reinforces these messages."[32] However, despite programs visually reinforcing the necessity of discipline, surveillance, and transformation, these programs also counter those same persuasive visual messages in two ways. First, the narratives and personal histories previously discussed, which make participants relatable or identifiable as opposed to mere objects for critique or derision, may undermine the shaming aspects of reality television while playing up the empathic aspects of such scenes. Second, the remainder of each episode regularly and inadvertently demonstrates that submitting oneself to the surveilling gaze of the camera, viewers at home, and each show's "experts" is not necessarily effective for sustained weight loss, weight maintenance, or developing self-control over one's body. In fact, shows like *Heavy* and *I Used to Be Fat* focus more on how challenging it is to lose weight and sustain that weight loss long term. Even if participants submit to constant surveillance in a controlled environment like those on *Heavy*'s Hilton Head Island resort, or allow a personal trainer to take control over their lives for three months like on *I Used to Be Fat*, losing weight—if weight is lost at all—is often shown to be a slow, difficult, and ongoing process.

Disciplinary Discrepancies and Weight-Loss Woes

Las Vegas is considered a city that never sleeps, so *Extreme Weight Loss* cameras follow Christy during a night out on the strip with her friends. At the end of the night, Christy pulls into a drive-through for a cheeseburger, explaining to the camera, "The one thing you can always count on is fast food." However, Powell interrupts her late-night snack to surprise her with the "transformation of her life," but only if she meets him on top of the Stratosphere before sunrise. The problem: it's a mile away and a 112-story climb to the top. Cameras follow Christy as she works her way down the street while she explains the difficulty of this journey, "I feel like I'm going to throw up right now and I haven't even climbed any stairs yet." But she continues, climbing step after step despite her labored breathing and perspiring through her shirt. She calculates that she needs to do a flight of stairs every minute in order to make it on time to be "chosen" for the series. After a dramatic pause on the 111th story, Christy successfully completes her first challenge. These types of challenges and other initial boot-camp-style workouts are meant to demonstrate the necessity of individuals losing weight, how "far they've let themselves go," and how difficult the journey will be. During Christy's first ninety days in the program, while living at a weight-loss facility in Colorado, she loses eighty-five pounds, almost one pound per day.

While the beginning of each episode (or season in the case of *The Biggest Loser*) does work along the same narrative lines as other makeover programs, the remainder of each episode is where narrative tension is built, and thus also where disciplinary discrepancies occur. According to most of the trainers on weight-loss programs, initial workouts are designed to show individuals just how "out of shape" they may be, but they can also undermine the rhetoric of health as actually being the goal of these programs. On *I Used to Be Fat* and *Extreme Weight Loss* participants are regularly shown becoming physically ill (vomiting, passing out, crying) due to the strenuous physical demands placed on them by TV trainers. Marci, a participant on *I Used to Be Fat*, says, "I'm going to pass out," and later, "I think I'm going to throw up." To these statements, her trainer only responds, "Alright, go throw up. You better throw up. Otherwise we're running." While the camera follows Marci to her spot lying on the bathroom floor next to the toilet, the trainer adds, "Marci if you don't get up out of that stall, I'm leaving and you can stay fat!" Alyssa, a season 3, episode 9 participant on *Extreme Weight Loss*, also collapses during her first workout, crying, "Everything hurts!" And forty days into the program she still either fights the urge to vomit or does vomit during her morning workouts. Powell attributes this to her body detoxing from her former diet of primarily fast food (for forty days?!). To "prove" to Alyssa the harm of her former diet, Chris decides to consume nothing but McDonald's and donuts until he also vomits. Similarly, contestants on *The Biggest Loser* are regularly shown becoming physically ill due to the strenuous physical demands placed on them by their TV trainers. For example, the first workout for the eighth season premiere results in the hospitalization of two contestants, Tracey and Mozziz. Tracey's hospital stay ends up lasting ten days, with sources reporting she was treated for rhabdomyolysis, a potentially fatal condition where overexerted muscles break down and release kidney-damaging proteins.[33]

There are numerous other weight-loss complications experienced by participants across these programs, including food temptations, exercise burnout, juggling careers and families with their exercise demands, lingering or developing emotional and mental health issues, and lacking familial support, all of which regularly result in weight-loss plateaus or even weight gain. According to Weber, makeover programs situate participants' "roller coaster of emotions" as something that must be contained in order to maintain progress.[34] Looking at contestants of *The Swan* (2004–2005) specifically, Weber argues that the ones who are "ungrateful, recalcitrant, resistant, or just negative are relentlessly portrayed as difficult."[35] Yet she also notes that these television narratives are used to create dramatic tension and "introduce the possibility that the makeover might fail."[36] On weight-loss series, the possibility of "failure" isn't just introduced by these shows; degrees of "failure" are regularly experienced by participants and exhibited on our television screens. These "failures" are productive in the sense that they protest (whether intrinsically or explicitly) the disciplinary techniques used by weight-loss TV programs.

These failures often occur even while participants are under constant surveillance. On early seasons of *Extreme Weight Loss* not only are cameras installed in all of the participants' homes, but Powell also allegedly moves in to provide them with 24/7 support and monitoring,[37] yet that does not prevent many of them from straying from their prescribed diet and exercise plans. A fairly common scene on *Extreme Weight Loss* is of participants sitting on their exercise equipment while eating and/or watching television. These scenes, as well as negative reports back from local trainers or private investigation teams following participants who stop communicating with Powell, are used to create suspense over whether the weight-loss transformation will be successful during the second and third phases of the program. Furthermore, they trouble assumptions about the effectiveness of surveillance to influence behavior. Cameras, impending weigh-ins, and surveillance teams do not translate to consistent discipline and sustained weight loss.

These programs also trouble television's role in teaching audiences self-discipline through the internalization of surveillance and disciplinary logics displayed on-screen. On more than one episode of *Heavy*, after three months of constant surveillance at a fitness facility (where participants lose all of their phone and television privileges and are limited in which personal belongings they have access to), participants like Tom and Rickywayne are still unable to sustain their weight-loss goals at home or choose to discontinue working out and dieting. Tom actually gains thirty pounds back during his first few weeks away from the facility. This weight gain then necessitates that participants return to an environment of constant surveillance and discipline at the weight-loss facility. These "failures" mean that they did not internalize the surveilling gaze or that the gaze was quickly "forgotten" once it was (partially) removed. Thus, even under surveillance, participant behavior does not always match "expert" expectations or follow "expert" directives.

Across numerous episodes of *I Used to Be Fat*, participants also fail to lose weight despite the help of "experts" and constant surveillance. One person featured on the show, Daria (season 1, episode 6), loses only a few pounds after a summer's worth of six-hour-a-day workouts. Even though Daria is monitored and held "accountable" by both her personal trainer and MTV viewers, her progress is disrupted by her mother, who continues to buy "junk foods" for the rest of the family and repeatedly tells Daria both that she does not have a "weight problem" and needs to work out less in order to contribute to the family financially. Daria's mother is positioned as an adversary to the trainer, but at the same time this situation complicates the efficiency or realistic possibility of entirely submitting oneself to the constant effort required by these TV programs, and at times almost frames such intense focus on the self as a selfish endeavor.

Despite having a personal trainer for about ninety days, many of the participants on *I Used to Be Fat* also struggle to meet their weight-loss goals. For example, Lindsey (season 2, episode 3) narrates her struggles during the second week of filming, "I just feel like I don't have enough hours in the day to do everything I have to do and it's really hard to get my homework done and get my workouts in and everything else that goes along with it." After three more weeks of near daily intensive training under the guidance of Ary, Lindsey has not lost any additional weight, which demonstrates the way the body itself can resist our efforts (or the way our efforts can result in bodily responses counter to weight-loss goals). When Latrice (season 2, episode 4) loses only a couple of pounds in the first two weeks of her training routine on *I Used to Be Fat* during the time when many participants drop significant weight, Latrice feels dejected and relaxes her

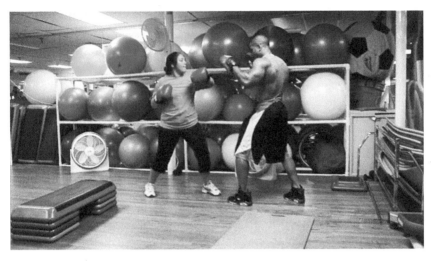

Figure 10   Lindsey on season 2 of *I Used to Be Fat* (2011)

eating habits. At one point, Latrice says to her trainer, "I haven't met any of my goals. I suck." Her trainer responds that it's a matter of effort and that he is *trying* to teach her self-discipline and accountability, but instead feels like he is just wasting his time. After thirty days of training with minimal "success," Latrice starts seeing a counselor to work through why she might be "self-sabotaging" her weight loss through her eating habits. With the help of two "expert" interventions, Latrice loses just a small amount of weight out of the one hundred pounds she planned to lose during the span of 105 days. However, neither her trainer nor the show's informational cards, which normally detail the progress of participants' weight-loss journeys by showing their original weights, goal weights, and weight loss since their last weigh-in, specify her total loss amount. Instead, *I Used to Be Fat* depicts the happiness of her family while narrating that Latrice now weighs 226 pounds and is "happy," which deemphasizes her minimal weight loss and the "failure" of the show itself. When the cameras catch up with her two months later at a poetry reading and audition, she still has not lost additional weight despite learning the "tools" to do so from her trainer, her counselor, and MTV.

Furthermore, on the final episode of season 1 of *I Used to Be Fat*, several of the participants are shown having gained weight back, including Gabriella and McKenzie. McKenzie even says about "maintaining" her body weight, "I'm not going to lie, it's really hard." In addition to the almost expected post-show weight gain, other participants barely finish, quit, or are "fired" from weight-loss programs just like on *Revenge Body*. Tanner, a season 1, episode 8 participant on *I Used to Be Fat*, loses thirty-seven pounds of his one-hundred-pound goal but gradually becomes unmotivated to lose more because he no longer wants to spend all of his free time working out. Ty (season 4, episode 1) on *Extreme Weight Loss* ultimately quits the program after a failed baseball deal and turns down an offer of "living" with Powell in Arizona to instead stay near his family and go back to his pre-show life.

A major weight-loss "failure" can also be seen in season 10 of *The Biggest Loser* where all of the contestants temporarily "join" the Marines. When the contestants are first told they will be training with the military, *The Biggest Loser* host, Alison Sweeney, explains to them, "You are halfway through the season, and you should be proud of how far you've come, but if you thought the first six weeks were a battle, this next week is going to be an all-out war." While highlighting the strenuous and difficult nature of the week ahead, this statement also implicitly downplays the effectiveness of *The Biggest Loser*'s intervention and training practices. One contestant, Jesse, similarly and unintentionally downplays his first six weeks at *The Biggest Loser* ranch while privileging the power of the military: "We all still have the mindset of 'Hey, I'm the fat guy. I can't cut it with the Marines.' This might be kind of the kick start we need." This statement implies that *The Biggest Loser*'s initial boot-camp-style workout was perhaps inefficient at maintaining discipline or garnering big weight-loss numbers long term.

The Marines episode also features contestants simultaneously engaging in strenuous physical activity and making "poor" food decisions during the week they are living on the base, which shows that the discipline they experienced the first six weeks on the show did not translate into self-disciplined eating decisions. Furthermore, the Marine base as a disciplinary site is also framed as not being conducive for weight loss. One contestant, Jesse, even states, "Here at the mess hall the options are not the options we would have at the ranch. Sausage. French toast. I anticipate a very grueling workout today and I decided I need the calories." Later, during the usual end-of-episode weigh-in, another contestant, Lisa, complains, "Eating in the mess hall . . . high sodium food. It hinders weight loss. We just had very little control over the food that we ate this week," and another, Elizabeth, laments, "I don't know what happened because I did put in the work. I gave it my all. The only thing I can say is we had no control over our own food. We couldn't measure things and that's the only thing I can think of." In fact, many of contestants fail to lose weight as temporary Marines and several actually gain weight, including Frado, a former Marine, who gains four pounds over the course of the week. As the week's weigh-in scene plays out, all of the trainers and contestants seem baffled as to how their experience as Marines did not translate into big weight-loss numbers.

Palmer contends that surveillance on weight-loss programs offers proof that an "increase in surveillance is effective in that nearly everyone loses weight and becomes happier," adding that this "recommends the technology as valuable in modern life."[38] Yet all of the examples discussed thus far emphasize that not everyone loses weight or becomes happier. Palmer does acknowledge a second, contradictory aspect of surveillance, namely that it "cannot be present all the time and thus leaves the contestants potentially susceptible to slipping back into old ways."[39] And even when surveillance is always present (like when participants join the Marines on *The Biggest Loser* or when the producers of *Extreme Weight Loss* install cameras in the homes of participants), some participants still do not exercise or eat as directed, turning treadmills into seats for television watching, as noted before. Again, many weight-loss shows portray participants as "likely susceptible," instead of "potentially susceptible," which also downplays TV's disciplinary role while playing up narrative tension.

Returning to Christy's story on *Extreme Weight Loss*, during her three-month weigh-in Powell warns her about the difficulties of phase 2 because that's "where real life starts pouring back in." Upon Christy returning from her boot camp in Colorado to begin the second phase, cameras are also installed in her newly converted workout space to monitor her activity and, of course, to capture B-roll in the absence of a camera crew. Despite the presence of cameras, Christy does not see continued progress toward her weight-loss goals. In fact, one month living at her surveilled home results in a three-pound weight gain instead of a double-digit loss. Powell, frustrated by her "always wanting to be the victim," decides to confront her at home. During the confrontational scene, Powell speculates that the gain is likely a result of portion issues or her not working out with enough intensity, but Christy is insulted by Powell even being there, saying, "I would have loved for you to have that validation that I'm in here stuffing my face on the couch, but that's not my reality at all. I'm not an overeater. I don't do all those things that got me where I was." Cutting away to an interview, Powell sarcastically says to the camera, "I'm sorry, but if this is true, if her nutrition is spot-on and she's doing four hours of exercise a day she shouldn't be doing a transformation with me she should be in a NASA space lab because she defies the laws of physics." Powell tells Christy she's moving back to Colorado, and she begrudgingly agrees despite worrying this means she will be unable to achieve her goals "on her own," meaning without Powell but still while under the surveillance of the show.

However, before Powell and Christy return to Colorado, Heidi (Powell's wife and fellow trainer on *Extreme Weight Loss*) confronts Christy while she's packing her belongings for the trip back to Colorado. Heidi says in an interview scene, "Before Chris and I bring Christy back to Colorado it's important that she admits she has not been following the plan that Chris and I set out for her. She can't shed the weight if she's holding on to a lie." Christy, instinctually, says to Heidi, "I don't cheat." Doubting this answer, Heidi asks, "So you haven't gone out with your girlfriends, drinking and doing all the stuff you used to do? At all?"

CHRISTY: Nope. I'm not drinking beer; I don't go through the fast-food drive-through, I don't get the big soda. . . .

HEIDI: Not once?

CHRISTY: Not once.

HEIDI: That's just not realistic to me. Period.

CHRISTY: I mean, what are you trying to get at because you're trying to put words in my mouth and it's not going to happen.

HEIDI: I'm not trying to put any words in your mouth. . . .

CHRISTY: I'm not going to tell you that I've been cheating. Period.

HEIDI: I just want you to be honest.

CHRISTY: Why do you keep pushing at it when I'm telling you to your face and God. I am not cheating.

HEIDI: I've never met a person in four seasons that has not slipped up along the way . . . my take, Christy, is that you're scared to go to Colorado because you know you're going to have to work hard and you're not ready to do that. I can feel it.

The scene cuts to Heidi again speaking directly to the camera, "If Christy doesn't change her attitude I'm worried she's not going to be able to do this at all." The show then cuts to Christy also addressing this exchange directly to the camera, "I want to lose the weight. I'm trying to lose the weight. I know what works and I don't understand what I'm doing wrong. If you have this plan and it's supposed to work, then why isn't it working for me?" It remains unclear to viewers whether Christy has actually been "cheating," as the show does not exhibit any footage of her out with her friends or eating more than her recommended diet. This lack of footage is particularly interesting because the show typically goes to great lengths to capture evidence of other participants who falter during phases 2 and 3 (a typical scenario on the show).

The next scene depicts Christy struggling to run hills back in Colorado. Powell gives her a pep talk and tells her to reflect on her commitment to transformation during her walk back to the Colorado campus. The next scene cuts to grainy black-and-white footage (captured by "Security Camera 3") showing Christy getting into a mysterious white car. We learn in the next scene that Christy is "hitchhiking" from the park back to the dorms. Both Heidi and Chris view this as a "final straw" and decide that she's not ready for their program. Powell says to the camera, "Christy is full of excuses. She wants to be the victim and doesn't want to work. If she truly wants transformation, she has to fight for it and she has to fight for it right now." He then says to Christy, "I need to know why you're here. . . . We all invested so much in you and you cheated yourself. Not only do you not believe in yourself, but you don't want to believe in yourself. Nothing is going to change until you make that committed decision." Heidi chimes in,

"Everybody wants this for you. Everybody does. Except for you. You need to go back home." Chris and Heidi subsequently hand Christy a plane ticket. She neither resists nor challenges what they're saying. In fact, she *wants* to go home, explaining, "There is a part of me that is relieved. I didn't know it was going to be as hard as it was. I had no idea." An off-camera producer then asks her, "Did you sabotage this on purpose?" Christy simply nods in response.

While these examples can be interpreted as personal failures on behalf of the participants, they can also be seen as failures of the shows themselves to effectively surveil and implement a body intervention for the purposes of transformation. These shows indeed follow a similar narrative structure to other makeover programs, but the makeovers themselves are more fraught with complications and, overall, are less likely to end with the reveal of an "after-body." This is likely the result of one of the major differences in weight-loss makeovers compared to others: the amount of work required by participants themselves. On weight-loss TV participants are required to engage in constant physical activity and calorie restriction in order to "transform." This kind of physical and emotional work is not required of participants redoing their wardrobes or home décor. And even when participants do the *work*—even when they submit to "expert" surveillance— sometimes the body itself does not cooperate in the transformation.

The Failures of "Eat Less and Do More!"

While these examples demonstrate that weight loss is neither constant nor predictable, despite conventional wisdom dictating our weights as being determined by calories in versus calories out, reunion episodes and follow-up reports on blogs and in news stories further demonstrate the fallacy of such discourses. Not only do these discourses surrounding weight-loss programs show the ephemerality and/or nonexistence of the "after-body" state, they also simultaneously expose the futility in submitting oneself to three months of constant surveillance and the inconsistencies of internalizing that state of being over the long term. One former contestant from season 2 of *The Biggest Loser*, Suzanne Mendonca, argues that the reason NBC never does a reunion (despite doing two carefully crafted reunion episodes in seasons 8 and 12) is that "we're all fat again!"[40] For example, the first season winner of *The Biggest Loser*, Ryan Benson, regained all of the weight he lost on the show. The show itself concedes that 50 percent of its participants do regain most of the weight they lose, if not more.[41]

The "Where Are They Now?" episodes and follow-up or reunion shows for other weight-loss series demonstrate that surveillance logics are not necessarily internalized and expert "interventions" may not have long-lasting impacts. An eighth season episode of *The Biggest Loser* features the first reunion episode of the series and visits forty contestants from the first seven seasons of the show to find out, according to trainer Jillian Michaels, "who is struggling, who kept it off, and who gained it all back. . . . No one said it would be easy!" Of course, a majority of the former contestants featured on this episode are success stories because it would be contrary to *The Biggest Loser*'s interests otherwise. However, the inclusion of unsuccessful past contestants illustrates the tension between the show needing to frame itself as an effective weight-loss intervention serving the public interest and its need to create dramatic or suspenseful narratives drawing viewers to the show. The inclusion of past participants who regain weight is also likely necessary because of increased criticism over the series' health practices across numerous news reports and blog posts, which I discuss in the concluding chapter. Defending the show, Mallory, who becomes a health trainer following her participation on *The Biggest Loser*, counters pervasive weight-gain rumors, "I just want to tell everybody that *The Biggest Loser* works!" Yet Matt and Suzy, who meet as contestants and later marry, both gain a considerable amount of weight back. Matt says to the camera during an interview, "You can tell by seeing us that we've gained some weight back." Suzy says, "You have to work at it and we're no different."

Also documented on this episode as well as another reunion episode in the show's tenth season are past winners who regain all of their lost weight. Erik gains 175 pounds after being on the show, returning within 40 pounds of his pre-*Loser* weight of 407 (his experience even inspired an episode of Discovery Health and Fitness's *Confessions of a Reality Show Loser* [2010]). When Bob Harper, a longtime trainer and later host of *The Biggest Loser*, visits him and asks him to explain his weight gain, Erik replies, "I got really low . . . and I started to just say fuck it." Erik then details his plan to return to the strict life he led while on *The Biggest Loser*, but Harper rather interestingly responds to him, "You can't go back to the strict life. You have to find balance to live the rest of your life. You can't do the extreme. You have to find a day-to-day life, what is going to work for you." This advice undermines the extreme logics of *The Biggest Loser*, which understandably confuses Erik and makes him question, "But how will I see results?" Similarly, Ryan, who regains almost all of the weight he lost while on *The Biggest Loser* ranch, believes that his weight gain was the result of not translating his habits from the strict environment on the ranch to his post-ranch life. Ryan does not elaborate on whether he just did not want to or could not pragmatically continue working out for several hours each day.

Other past participants not featured on "Where Are They Now?" episodes have also opened up about regaining weight post–*The Biggest Loser*. Ali Vincent, a season 5 winner (and the first woman to win) gained back almost all of the 112 pounds she lost. Vincent says she continued to use a calorie counter after the show and "childproofed her life" so as "not to leave anything to guesswork," yet still gained weight.[42] Vincent discusses the shame she feels—and her inability to even get out of bed on the eighth anniversary of her win—in an OWN series, *Where Are They Now*, saying, "The truth is I kind of spiraled. I got home and I was like 'what do I do? What do I do without the ranch?'"[43] Kate Hibbard, a season 3 participant, also details stories of self-dehydration and working out in multiple layers of clothes to lose more weight for the weekly weigh-in. As a result of these practices, Hibbard says she gained thirty-one pounds just by drinking water during her first two weeks away from the show.[44] The winner of season 8, Danny Cahill, reportedly regained a hundred of the almost two hundred pounds he lost, with most of his colleagues on that season gaining all of their lost weight back (with some now weighing more than they did at the start of the show).[45]

While *The Biggest Loser* and *Extreme Weight Loss* do contain the most fat-to-thin transformations, *I Used to Be Fat* primarily features participants who, although unable to reach their weight loss goals, are nevertheless happy in their still larger-than-desired bodies. *Heavy* typically ends with most participants still weighing three to four hundred pounds, preferring the goal of a much more gradual weight loss than its more spectacularized counterparts. Again, these examples attest to the somewhat empty promise of television to discipline the bodies on-screen and viewers' bodies at a distance, revealing the faulty logics of the surveilling gaze in a society of discipline and control. Even though contestants are willing to submit themselves to the trainers' and viewers' constant monitoring and are taught by "experts" how to self-discipline, "success" is never guaranteed and is infrequently achieved.

In fact, as the episode or season endings, follow-up episodes, academic studies, and public criticism attest, these weight-loss series never lead to a final "after," and few of them result in scenes revealing the participants' desired after-body. Normally, the reveal scene is when participants earn the *privilege* of being clothed; even if they do not make it to their goal weights, they are portrayed as now being "fully human" and as having the appearance of their outside selves compatible with their inside selves. Like the initial weigh-ins, reveal scenes are often public and occur before large audiences. Weber explains the logic of these scenes: "Structuring the reveals in ways that require external validation (as corroborated by enthusiastic doctors, supportive friends, self-evaluations in a mirror, or interpellated viewer approval) confers a ratifying power in spectatorial surveillance, affirming the rightness" of the transformation.[46] Yet as Martin Roberts points out, "To date lifestyle television has produced little evidence that its transformative magic lasts any longer than the day on which it takes place."[47]

Additionally, "successful" reveals themselves can backfire in supporting both TV and common weight-loss logics. After fifteen seasons of "helping" contestants lose weight, these controversial aspects of *The Biggest Loser* are getting even more attention. Rapid weight loss, low-calorie diets, and rumors of diuretic use or fasting before weigh-ins undermine claims made by both the show's fitness trainers and contestants, who frame their actions and participations as being primarily in service of health. The conclusion of the fifteenth season, in particular, gave these issues broader attention as the winner, Rachel Frederickson, lost one hundred fifty pounds in seven months. Her transformation reclassified her, according to the BMI, as also going from super or morbidly obese to under-weight, raising questions regarding not only the show's tactics and motives, but also the parameters for what types of bodies are deemed healthy.

During her body reveal and final weigh-in, trainer Jillian Michaels's jaw literally dropped upon seeing Rachel's new, small frame, which was described in news reports as "emaciated."[48] Headlines the following day read, "'Biggest Loser' Win-ner: Too Thin?," "Shamed for Being Fat, Then for Being Thin," and "'Biggest Loser' Winner Rachel Frederickson Says She May Have Gone Too Far."[49] While thinness is undoubtedly still aesthetically idealized and often medically pre-scribed, this example of bodies being problematic if they are perceived as either too fat or too thin illustrates the impossible bodily constraints and pressures that women in particular face, and also a potential turning point in the way thin bod-ies tend to be uncritically praised and automatically linked with conceptualiza-tions of good health. While these narratives may be shifting, or exposing flaws in widely accepting weight-loss logics, and in weight-loss TV programs, the prem-ise that weight loss is desirable and necessary for health remains, at least for the most part, intact.

Conclusion

The Biggest Loser is frequently accused of putting "entertainment before health,"[50] and I argue that it also puts television's role as an entertainer before its role as a discipliner at a distance, despite Roth's claims about the show operating in the public interest. Further, some studies suggest that instead of motivating people to exercise and eat better—the public service identified by Roth—watchers of *The Biggest Loser* are less inclined to want to exercise.[51] This is because of the way exercise is represented, according to Tanya Berry: "People are screaming and crying and throwing up, and if you're not a regular exerciser you might think this is what exercise is—that it's this horrible experience where you have to push yourself to the extremes and the limits, which is completely wrong."[52]

By playing up the tension between trainers and participants and focusing as much on weight-loss plateaus, weight gains, and emotional stories as on trans-formational "successes," these series complicate simplistic yet dominant assump-tions about fatness and the logics of weight-loss TV by showing that eating less and moving more mostly fails at changing the size of bodies both on- and off-camera. These shows inadvertently push back against notions that fatness is merely the result of gluttony or laziness yet reinforce the notion that being fat is an undesirable bodily state. These series, according to Dr. Huizinga (season 8, episode 12), reduce stigma by showing that it's okay to be fat and work out (and maybe that people can be fat *and* fit?), yet still suggests that six- to eight-hour daily workouts are the "answer" to fat embodiment.

Even though programs like *Extreme Weight Loss* focalize particular discourses of fatness because of various industrial, regulatory, and aesthetic forces that influence the way stories are told and how people are represented on the small screen, TV often undermines the very discourses it articulates and recirculates. Television programs, then, simultaneously reflect and reinforce, as well as negotiate and challenge, globally circulated discourses of the fat body in the context of the obesity epidemic. These shows represent fatness as a choice, but they also undermine the *actual* ability for us to simply choose the size of our bodies through exercise and diet and television's ability to facilitate those choices and transformations.

6 Spectacle, Sympathy, and the Medicalized Disease of "Obesity"

In the fall of 2016, BBC3 aired a controversial documentary special titled *Obesity: The Post-Mortem*. The show frames itself as educational, as examining through an autopsy of anonymous fat woman the "hidden effects" of obesity on the body, effects only the body itself can reveal after death to pathologists and viewers at home. The autopsy takes place in a darkly lit room with only the naked body visible as the camera pans over the woman's pale and blistering flesh while pathologists remove and dissect her organs. Some viewers describe this television documentary as "necessary" or "boundary-pushing," and others read it as being "a fatphobic freak show."[1] Critics viewed it, at its worst, as cruel, and, at its best, as ineffective at "halting the obesity epidemic."[2] Regardless of whether *Obesity: The Post-Mortem* is necessary or cruel, boundary-pushing or fatphobic, it functions much like other televised spectacles of medicine or fatness: attempting to scare or shame viewers at home into assessing their own bodies and medical statuses. This "spectacle of shame" thus positions the fat body as a site of failure that allows us to "revel in the spectacle of the grotesque body."[3] Yet while the televised medical gaze may, indeed, be shaming and controlling as it is in *Obesity: The Post-Mortem*, it may also foster compassion and understanding in other television contexts.[4]

With bright lights, elaborately constructed scales for weigh-ins, tension-filled narratives, and dramatic performances, exercise and diet-based shows like *The Biggest Loser* can be considered television spectacles.[5] However, this chapter focuses on the framing of the fat body itself as a spectacle and examines a different kind of relationship between television and spectacle due to the medicalized framing of fatness as the disease of obesity. The TLC program *My 600-lb Life* (2012–) and its follow-up spinoff *My 600-lb Life: Where Are They Now?* (2014–) both emphasize the *struggle* to lose weight via "heart wrenching journeys of addiction, shame, and determination."[6] *My 600-lb Life* began filming in 2004 as a documentary miniseries following four participants over the course of seven years, but in the show's second season, beginning in 2012, each participant is followed over a one-year period with updates provided by the spin-off series. The fact that this show borrows more heavily from the documentary tradition and frames itself as more observational than reality shows in the makeover or even game show subgenres influences how we make sense of what we're seeing on-screen.[7] The show presents itself as not intervening in fatness; rather it's just capturing the story of a fat intervention. There is no host, only minimal narration through subtitling and on-screen text. There are no food or elimination challenges or brightly lit workout rooms, only shots of participants in their homes, hospitals, and vehicles as they travel between their homes and hospitals. While the distinctions between documentary and reality TV are somewhat arbitrary (because they rely on malleable extratextual discourses and specific cultural practices),[8] they do encourage us to see the representations and narratives as socially important or educational rather than as sensational or exploitative. And this has important implications for how we understand both fatness and spectacularized images of the body.

Unlike the weight-loss series discussed in chapter 5, these programs represent a shift away from the dominant narrative of fatness televised within the obesity epidemic. Instead of fatness positioned as a lifestyle choice or the result of lacking personal responsibility, willpower, or self-control, medicalized fat television focuses on the fat body as both a complex medical issue and the disease of obesity. Although this chapter focuses on *My 600-lb Life*, numerous other medicalized shows frame fatness in similar ways, including *I Eat 33,000 Calories a Day* (2007), *Big Medicine* (2007–), *Inside Brookhaven Obesity Clinic* (2007–), *Half-Ton Teen* (2009), *Embarrassing Bodies* (2010–), *My Deadly Appetite* (2010), *World's Fattest Man* (2010), *Britain's Fattest Man* (2010), *I'm Eating Myself to Death* (2010), *Fat Doctor* (2007–2012), *650 Pound Virgin* (2012), *Obese & Expecting* (2012–), *The Real Skinny* (2012–2013), and many others that primarily circulate in the United States, the United Kingdom, Canada, and Australia.

After first discussing television's pro-medicine history and the mutually reinforcing medicalizations of fatness, television, and society more broadly, the goal of this chapter is twofold: first, I demonstrate how the experiences of fatness represented on *My 600-lb Life* through the framing of fatness as a disease, rather than as just an individual failing, positions fat individuals in a way that also fosters sympathy, compassion, and potentially other kinds of "affective investment,"[9] rather than just disciplining, shaming, or acting as a "warning" to viewers at home. As discussed previously, most literature on reality television transformations focuses on lifestyle television and cosmetic makeovers. These shows present bodies as unruly or abject and then controllable or governable once they submit to surveillance and are transformed.[10] But transformation takes on additional meaning when it's characterized by medicalized discourses of disease, when it's deemed necessary for just staying alive. Whereas assumptions that we have control over the size of our bodies leave little to no room for bodily sympathy, at least according to some,[11] shows like *My 600-lb Life* mitigate the assigning of personal blame for fat embodiment by framing fatness as a disease rather than a lifestyle choice. This creates space for sympathy at least as much as it fosters bodily shame. Second, I argue that these representations of fatness as the disease of obesity offer a competing narrative that complicates "common sense" assumptions regularly perpetuated by weight-loss reality television by instead reinforcing the necessity of medical authority over the fat body and medical treatments for fatness. Yet these shows are similarly fraught with contradictions, tensions, and failures of bodily intervention and transformation.

The Medical Gaze and Medicalized Television

In order to understand the uniqueness of contemporary medicalized representations of fatness, we need to think about the relationships between medicine and bodies as well as between medicine and television. In *The Birth of the Clinic* (1963), Foucault describes the "medical gaze" to explain how the body becomes an object of the gaze for observing and diagnosing, where medicine constitutes patients and dehumanizes individuals, separating patients from their bodies and disciplining and categorizing bodies according to medical discourses as either normal or pathological, healthy or unhealthy. Foucault also details hospitals and clinics as specific sites for exerting this disciplinary power and for the emergence of "general disciplinary technologies."[12] The medicalization of society and emergence of disciplinary technologies allow medical authority to transcend the institutional space of the hospital or the clinic to discipline society at large.[13] Nikolas Rose argues that medicine is now a matter of assemblages or combinations of spaces, persons, and techniques. These assemblages include what Rose refers to as "five apparatuses of health," which are intertwined with and shape our daily lives in numerous ways, including the "medical administration of public spaces" and "hygienic regulations of domestic life."[14] Medicalized television, indeed, acts as another apparatus of health, or another part of the broader social "medical assemblage" because it further expands medical authority and medical knowledge outside of the walls of hospitals and clinics through television content.[15]

Not only is the authority of the hospital or clinic as a site of discipline dispersed throughout a society of control via television and Rose's other apparatuses of health, but that dispersal reinforces the authority and disciplinary status of those institutions. During the 1970s there was also a rise in what Julie Elman refers to as "medicalized edutainment." Elman argues that during that time there was an increase of television content intending to "digest, transmit, and construct images of medical knowledge and often disability for public consumption, entertainment, and education."[16] In fact, medical storylines across soap operas were once so common that George Gerbner and colleagues speculated, "It may well be that daytime serials are the largest source of medical advice in the United States."[17] Prime-time television also consistently featured and continues to feature medical doctors and medical storylines, including shows such as *City Hospital* (1951–1953), *Medic* (1954–1956), *Dr. Kildare* (1961–1966), *Ben Casey* (1961–1966), *Medical Center* (1969–1976), *Emergency!* (1972–1979), *Marcus Welby M.D.*

(1969–1976), *St. Elsewhere* (1982–1988), *Doogie Howser, M.D.* (1989–1993), *Dr. Quinn: Medicine Woman* (1993–1998), *ER* (1994–2009), *Chicago Hope* (1994–2000), *Gideon's Crossing* (2000–2001), *Scrubs* (2001–2010), *Presidio Med* (2002–2003), *Grey's Anatomy* (2005–), *Private Practice* (2007–2013), *House* (2004–2012), *Royal Pains* (2009–2016), *Nurse Jackie* (2009–2015), *Emily Owens, M.D.* (2012–2013), and many, many others.

Past medicalized television programs tended to represent the field and medical professionals positively. These positive portrayals are likely a result of already existent respect for medicine and its authority over the body, and undoubtedly contribute to the continuation of these sentiments among viewers. According to Joseph Turow, "Television's producers had no intention of creating programs that attack the legitimacy of the nation's health care professions. Doctors, especially, were the central heroes of TV medicine's struggle against death and it would be dramatically self-defeating to make them fundamentally unsympathetic."[18] Similarly, Gregory Makoul and Limor Peer contend that many medical television programs glamorize doctors and the health care system more generally.[19] These typical representations of the medical field reflect long-standing discourses of doctors as being "experts" not only of the body but also of the "art of living" more generally.[20] Even potentially unsympathetic doctors, like the strange and painkiller-addicted Gregory House on *House* and the strange and painkiller-addicted Jackie Peyton on *Nurse Jackie*, are still shown to be great healers and smart medical practitioners. Furthermore, historical representations of doctors and the field of medicine are at least partially influenced by the Physician Advisory Committee for Radio, Television, and Motion Pictures, which the American Medical Association developed in 1955. This committee consults on medical programs to *safeguard the credibility of physician portrayals* and medical knowledge circulated.[21] Marc R. Cohen and Audrey Shafer argue that there is a cyclical relationship between how fictional doctors are represented on television and how we view and interpret actual doctors off-screen. They maintain that medical doctors on television embody the same characteristics that viewers expect all heroic protagonists to embody, which makes doctors more likely to be represented as brilliant diagnosticians, as all-knowing across every medical subspecialty, and as always being able to cure patients.[22] As a result, at least according to Cohen and Shafer, we tend to frame non-TV doctors through the same heroic, talented, and knowledgeable lenses.

In addition to these representational trends across fictional programs throughout television's history, news reports, talk shows, made-for-TV documentaries, and reality programs all circulate medicalized understandings of the body. There was actually an entire cable channel devoted to such information in the mid-1990s, the American Medical Network (now part of FitTV), which had an agreement with the famous Mayo Clinic to draw on hospital resources for television content. The American Medical Network's president, Joe Maddox, stated during the network's development that in addition to the Mayo agreement, the network would feature live "Ask a Doctor" programs each day, featuring around twenty "telegenic physicians" as hosts.[23] According to Lester D. Friedman, these kinds of networks and other television programs become a major source of health care and medical information for the public.[24] Likewise and more specifically, Dorothy Nelkin argues that most people (including physicians!) get information about the potential medical risks of fatness from news media as opposed to reading academic or research-oriented scientific or medical publications.[25] Just as talk shows, news media, and medicalized television programs use medical stories for headlines and plots, the field of medicine relies on mediated texts to publicize research results, legitimize medical knowledge, and reinforce medical authority over the fat body. Concurrently, television aids in the medicalization of bodies by "helping" viewers consider themselves ill or at risk for illness and then offering them solutions that combine commercial interests with medical authority.[26]

Shows like *The Doctors* (2008–) and *Dr. Oz* (2009–), as well as segments across news broadcasts and day-time programs, such as *The Chew* (2011–), *The Today Show* (1952–), and *The View* (1997–), regularly discuss medical treatments for fatness. For example, one episode of *The Doctors* discusses abdominal fat, referred to by one scrub-wearing host as "toxic goop that increases inflammation . . . basically an alien invasion." Another host rhetorically asks and answers, "What happens when you get rid of belly fat? Studies show you'll actually be smarter, you'll sleep better, and you'll have a healthier heart." But wait, there's more! The host then explains that reductions in belly fat also lead to "better sex and even more money." The segment then transitions into a discussion and demonstration of liposuction for abdominal fat removal. A more extreme story about medical treatments for fatness occurs during the 2013 season of *Dr. Phil*. Dr. Phil pays for the bariatric surgery of an eight-hundred-pound man, Robert Gibbs, and his admittance to Wellspring Weight-Loss Academy. *Dr. Phil* cameras follow Gibbs's "success" over multiple episodes as the twenty-three-year-old man loses some of his eight hundred pounds under both medical and televisual supervision, "proving" that medical treatment is beneficial for even the most "extreme" fat bodies.

When the AMA classified obesity as a disease, which I discuss in chapter 2, numerous television programs, from nightly news reports to talk show segments, also discussed the implications of the label in addition to exploring medical treatments. A nightly news segment on CBS New York discussing the AMA's classification of obesity as a disease features Dr. Shawn Garber, director of the New York Bariatric Group, discussing weight-loss surgery as a good option for struggling individuals, an option now also more likely to be covered by insurance providers. A few years earlier, Dr. Garber made similar television appearances to discuss the Food and Drug Administration's decision to lower the weight threshold for Lap-Band surgery qualification, requiring that individuals can be just thirty pounds overweight to qualify as long as they have an "obesity-related disease."

Introducing the topic on *Dr. Oz* (April 4, 2013), Dr. Oz explains, "This could help twenty-five million more Americans lose the pounds and keep them off." Dr. Garber continues, "Now more than ever Lap-Band is a great option for patients. FDA data shows that 85 percent of patients were successful with the Lap-Band whereas regular diets show an over 85 percent failure rate." The discussion then expands to include two women in the audience who would now qualify for Lap-Band surgery given the lowered threshold. Both of them believe it would be a good option not only in terms of achieving weight loss, but also for *preventing* future "obesity-related diseases." One audience member explains to Dr. Oz, "The surgery, for me, is a good option to do something about it before I become morbidly obese." This segment thus "sells" weight-loss surgery to a larger group of smaller individuals, which happens to be the same group of individuals now classified as being diseased. It also reinforces the medicalized notion that bodies just presumed to be at risk for future illness are *already* considered ill or diseased and requiring of medical treatment. Now interspersed between headlines telling us to diet and exercise our ways to a slim physique are ones advising "Don't Put Off Weight Loss Surgery Until You're Heavier."

However, the same medicalized media that reinforce medical authority and treatments for weight loss are not always given the same positive framing as the medical doctors of television's past. For instance, analyses of the medical knowledge circulated by Dr. Oz, who is sometimes called "America's Doctor," indicate that less than a third of what he says on the show can be supported by even "modest medical evidence," and that four out of every ten of his medical claims have no basis in medical evidence.[27] Eventually, Dr. Oz was actually called before the U.S. Senate's consumer protection panel to defend his "miraculous" weight-loss supplement claims and recommendations of "revolutionary" treatments to viewers.[28] Shortly afterward, a nutrition expert featured on *Dr. Oz* reached a nine-million-dollar settlement with the Federal Trade Commission for falsely promoting the weight-loss power of a coffee supplement on television.[29] Similar skepticism over the validity of medical information on television circulated during the height of *Dr. Phil*, particularly as to whether he is actually a doctor (he does have a Ph.D.), and whether his television program constitutes practicing psychology without a license (technically, it does not).

The medicalization of bodies and the medicalization of television are mutually reinforcing trends. Television and other commercial entities are important vehicles for broad social medicalization, and medicalized television gains storylines, headlines, relevance, and social significance. This mutually reinforcing relationship is likely exacerbated by the "information overload" we experience thanks to social media, a twenty-four-hour news cycle, and the proliferation of cable channels in need of inexpensive and interesting content to fill their schedules.[30] Viewers are increasingly encouraged to migrate between multiple screens or media platforms, too. While watching *Dr. Oz*, viewers are encouraged to go to the show's website for more information about the fitness plans or "cancer fighting" recipes featured during TV segments. Numerous websites, mobile medical apps, and health tracking devices also exist to complement medicalized television programs or directly connect to them. Health-conscious TV viewers can track their calories or fitness levels on MyFitnessPal, check their symptoms on WebMD or AskMD, get reports of their heart rates and calories burned from Fitbit, and seek medical advice by calling Doctor On Demand, which is a service endorsed by *The Doctors*, all while being medically (mis)informed and hailed as potential patient-customers by the TV screen. There are about one hundred thousand mobile medical apps on the market that also allegedly screen for skin cancer, report on lung functioning, measure blood pressure and joint inflammation, and track menstrual cycles. Although all of these applications give users more data/info about their bodies than ever before, the questionable reliability of this information parallels the questionable advice disseminated by medicalized TV. Just as Dr. Oz is frequently referred to as a "Snake Oil Salesman,"[31] mobile medical apps are receiving criticism for their inaccuracy (Pfizer recalled its rheumatology calculator app after it was found to be inexact), for their lack of FDA regulation because they are categorized as "entertainment" or "informational" (medicalized edutainment) as opposed to medically diagnostic, and for potentially putting individuals in medical danger if they rely on these apps as opposed to medical authority.[32]

These apps, online forums, and medicalized television programs can also be used to spread awareness, challenge medical authority, and allow people to find support and share medical information and experiences. However, greater access to medical knowledge on TV and elsewhere may also make us more likely to believe we need medical treatment (regardless of whether we actually do), and therefore more likely to submit ourselves to medical monitoring or authority on or off television. Pessimistically, watchers of *Dr. Oz*, or readers of pharmaceutical advertisements found between the pages of magazines, may be more likely to view themselves as medicalized beings and inquire about and pay for unnecessary treatments and drugs to fix perceived problems, but optimistically, others may encounter those same messages and learn about potentially needed, beneficial treatments or options for care. This makes medical information more accessible to those of us outside the field of medicine, but it also positions us as perpetual patients.

The spread of medicalized information across medicalized television is ultimately important for differentiating between the framing of fatness as a disease and as a health choice. This, in turn, has important implications for the relationships between the spectacularized images of fatness that we see on our screens and television's role in disciplining, surveilling, and extending the medical gaze beyond the walls of the hospital or clinic. TV is of course complicit in positioning viewers as potential patients and in reproducing medical authority as it spreads medical knowledge, but frequently (even if inadvertently) TV also challenges that authority and knowledge. According to Deborah Lupton, "The existence of strategies of power does not necessarily correspond with the successful exertion of power, and . . . intended outcomes often fail to materialize because disciplinary strategies break down and fail."[33] Foucault himself encourages us to think about the ways in which power is productive as opposed to simply confining, saying, "power, after investing itself in the body, finds itself exposed to a counter-attack in the same body."[34] Thus, I argue that medicalized fat television is as inherently contradictory as the weight-loss television discussed in chapter 5. Fat bodies are repeatedly represented as diseased and in need of medical treatment, but the medicalized treatments typically featured rarely prove to be "successful," which complicates the legitimacy and perceived infallibility of medical authority over the body. Although the "medical-televisual gaze" is typically considered depersonalizing and objectifying,[35] through detailed personal stories and articulations to discourses of fatness as a disease, shows like *My 600-lb Life* complicate the relationship between spectacle and shame while creating space for spectacles of sympathy.

Bodily Spectacle and Sympathy

Spectacle can mean the public exhibition or display of someone or something by those in power.[36] Spectacle can also be in the form of surgical procedures on medicalized television that allow us to see inside of the body,[37] positioning spectacle as something that is shown or made visible for all to see, much like the previously discussed *Obesity: The Post-Mortem*. And it can also be understood in the Foucauldian sense, as in the spectacle of the scaffold working to "make an example, not only by making people aware that the slightest offense was likely to be punished, but by arousing feelings of terror by the spectacle of power letting its anger fall upon the guilty person."[38] While a spectacle could theoretically transform the "many-headed mob into an ordered crowd,"[39] Foucault notes that it was not uncommon for people to also reject this kind of punitive power, sometimes trying to thwart executioners or attempting to free prisoners, arguing, "It was evident that the great spectacle of punishment ran the risk of being rejected by the very people to whom it was addressed."[40] The resistance and revolts that Foucault details reminds us of the importance of considering the multiple ways in which we one can read or react to not only public events, but also what we see on our television screens, particularly spectacular exhibitions of the fat body.

Despite these different public interpretations of spectacle, we regularly think about the spectacle of reality television in terms of its disciplining or shaming potential.[41] Mediated medicalized spectacles, specifically, are thought to function primarily in terms of surveilling the body or gazing at the body, and thus controlling the body,[42] with the television camera providing the "vehicle for inspection."[43] In fact, David Lyon argues that spectacle is an important aspect of reality television because it "parades" the body in front of audiences.[44] Brenda Weber also considers the spectacular exhibition of "before-bodies" an important aspect of reality television that focuses on transformation, especially of the lifestyle makeover variety. For Weber, the display of before-bodies is meant to foster shame and to be evidence of "the subject's need for an intervention."[45] These before-bodies are thus positioned as deserving of ridicule and judgment, with fat individuals "regularly mocked as symbols of indulgence and moral decay" on weight-loss programs like *The Biggest Loser.*[46]

The display of bodies is considered a disciplinary feature across reality television, but like others who argue that shame and humiliation are not the only "affective drivers" of these programs, or that the televisual gaze can be both punishing and a source of pleasure and stimulation for viewers, I argue that spectacle functions differently on medicalized fat television framing fatness as a disease.[47] Indeed, Jeff Jervis points out that sympathy has long been implicated in spectacle, arguing that we as humans generally do not feel good about the suffering of others, but we do feel good about our "capacity to respond sympathetically *to* other's suffering."[48] For Jervis, the sympathy response is likely when a "basic dimension of human suffering comes into view" and when there are no questions of blame.[49] First, because participants in *My 600-lb Life* are portrayed to be suffering from physical impairment, social disability, or the prospect of being near death, fostering further shame through these experiences of fat embodiment via television could be read as unnecessarily cruel and exploitive. Tiara Sukhan argues that on the weight-loss program *The Last 10 Pounds Bootcamp* (2007) it is difficult to encourage "shame-inducing" disgust because participants are not considered medically obese.[50] But on *My 600-lb Life*, the same is true of the opposite: it's similarly difficult to encourage "shame-inducing" disgust precisely *because* participants are considered medically obese and *because* they are deemed in need of help beyond the health and lifestyle recommendations of diet and exercise. Second, across weight-loss television, fat individuals are regularly portrayed as suffering, but participants are almost always framed in terms of being personally responsible for their fatness (even if weight gain is contextualized as following the experience of a traumatic event, for example), or as being "to blame" for their bodies, but in the case of medicalized fat television, especially programs like *My 600-lb Life*, the notion of personal responsibility is negotiated because of the label of disease and corresponding stories of personal trauma, physical impairment, and social disability. Because the disease label potentially mitigates personal blame, in the sense that discourses of disease differ from the notion that fatness is the result of a character flaw or personal failing, I argue that it also alters television spectacle's function as shaming or disciplining to fostering sympathy, compassion, and similar types of affective investment.

My 600-lb Life: Televising Fatness as a Disease

"Food addiction has become my life. I let food be the way that I found solitude."
This narration is by Penny (season 2, episode 3), who weighs around six hundred
pounds and has been bedridden for several years. Introductory scenes depict
Penny's husband rubbing ointment between the folds of her exposed skin, while
she details her abusive childhood and its detrimental impact on her relationship
with food. Much like weight-loss reality television shows, each episode of *My
600-lb Life* begins this same way: participants discuss their histories and current
statuses while submitting their bodies to the gaze of the camera and to viewers
at home. Like Penny, Charity (season 3, episode 8) discusses her difficult childhood characterized by her alcoholic father, living in a constant state of panic,
and finding comfort in food. In the second episode of the fourth season of *My
600-lb Life*, Nikki details her history of fatness, namely the fact that she began
gaining weight around the age of four, that she weighed over one hundred forty
pounds by the age of ten, and that her parents tried "probably hundreds of
attempts" to help her lose weight. At thirty-three years old and six hundred pounds,
Nikki talks about both feeling trapped in her own body, although she retains
limited physical mobility, and feeling most at ease and comforted while eating.
Similarly, Brandi and Kandi, who are twins featured on the first episode of the
fifth season, detail their turbulent childhood and how their use of food to emotionally cope caused each of them to weigh two hundred pounds by middle
school and three hundred pounds by high school. Other participants on *My 600-lb
Life* detail experiences of trauma, food addiction, or depression as reasons for
gaining weight, with most saying they have been fat since childhood or puberty.
Whereas Palmer argues that "lifestyle formats that target the large" position
individual agency as "center stage, which makes any blame directed outside the
self seem weak,"[51] these stories on *My 600-lb Life* provide a more complex and
understandable backstory as to participants' current experiences of fat embodiment (not that unlike the stories discussed in chapter 5).

Similar to other weight-loss and makeover reality television programs, *My
600-lb Life* participants have their history supplemented with the visual surveilling or "diagnosing" of the naked fat body. As Weber and others argue, many
reality series foster shame by providing visual evidence that participants need an
intervention, or in this case medical treatment.[52] But on *My 600-lb Life* participants already feel shame over the size and appearance of their bodies (as Tara
says in season 2, "I'm disgusted by myself"), and they actively want medical
treatment. Further, while many reality programs of this nature "break down"
participants through surveillance that brings about humiliation before becoming
kinder and "knowing the subject more fully,"[53] on *My 600-lb Life* spectacular visu-
als are exhibited in tandem with personal narratives that frame fat embodiment
sympathetically or compassionately. Most participants are shown showering,

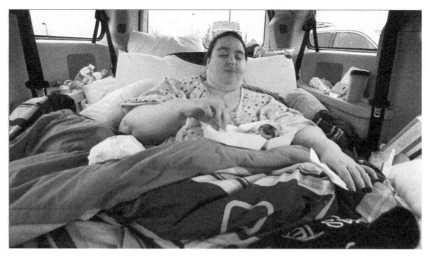

Figure 11   Penny being transported to the hospital on season 2 of *My 600-lb Life* (2014)

bathing, or being washed by their caregivers (typically romantic partners or family members) as they detail the difficulties of taking care of themselves because of the physical limitations of their size. For instance, the first line of diegetic dialogue in the eighth episode of the third season of *My 600-lb Life* is of Charity, who weighs 778 pounds, saying to her partner, "You gotta bring that toilet over, babe," because standard toilets are unable to hold someone of her size. On Brandi and Kandi's episode, they take turns showering, thoroughly cleaning between the folds of their flesh to prevent blisters while detailing the difficulty of shampooing their hair due to the heaviness of their arms. While the sisters take turns drying and powdering one another post-shower, Kandi says into the camera, "We're getting so big we can barely take care of each other. We still have to try because it's hard to do anything on our own." These scenes, while undoubtedly exploring each participant's bodily shame, also emphasize both the daily emotional and physical pain these individuals experience as they perform mundane daily tasks and the pervasive fear that they may not live much longer. This is compounded by Dr. Nowzaradan's generally "compassionate" approach to treating patients on the show;[54] he does not need to break them down before building them up like on *The Biggest Loser*—participants on *My 600-lb Life* are already framed as "broken."

In addition to these "private" moments re-created for television audiences at home, participants on *My 600-lb Life* who are able are then shown going out into public. Most of these public excursions revolve around food, whether depicting Kandi and Brandi going through a drive-through or Melissa (season 1, episode 1) utilizing a power scooter at a grocery store while other shoppers stare and comment on her weight. Participants universally talk about these socially disabling aspects of their fat embodiment: being stared at, overhearing negative comments and judgments, or strangers giving them unsolicited diet advice or weight-loss encouragement. If participants are physically impaired and bedridden, *My 600-lb Life* documents the foods that friends and family members bring into the home and the ways in which they "enable" and even encourage certain kinds of behavior. For example, Kandi and Brandi's mother brings them fast food—which is framed as an attempt to make up for their troubled childhoods—despite Kandi saying to the camera while crying, "I can't stop eating, but my weight is killing me. It's getting close to our final days." The combination of personal narratives of participants struggling to do ordinary activities like showering or grocery shopping and the visual excess of the fat body on the screen is consistent with what Douglas Kellner refers to as the "spectacle of everyday life."[55] Although spectacular images are not typically part of our everyday lives, Patricia Hughes-Fuller notes that with reality television the opposite seems to be true: everyday life is embedded in the context of spectacle.[56] I argue that this paradoxical combination of the spectacular and the mundane vis-à-vis medicalized fat television fosters sympathy as a form of affective engagement for audiences, if not more so, then as much as shame. As viewers we see the shame, embarrassment, and struggles participants *already* endure just to complete the most basic life tasks. Just lying in bed can be painful for some of the individuals featured on these shows. To frame these spectacularized bodies only in terms of shame without also framing individuals sympathetically would result in a particularly cruel form of television that might make viewers reject its punitive power.

The fat body at risk for disease, and thus already diseased, is continually reinforced across *My 600-lb Life* and numerous medicalized fat TV programs, which further work to foster sympathy for participants on the show. For example, Dr. Nowzaradan argues that Tara (season 2, episode 8) is at the point where she may not live for five more years because of her size. Although Tara and some other participants on the series never specify having any "obesity-related diseases," what matters most to the medicalized TV narrative and her bodily status is not that she could contract a disease, but rather that her weight means she already has. Of course being at risk for disease is not the only aspect of fatness explored; "obesity-related diseases" are a theme throughout many episodes, and in some ways are the focus of medicalized narratives of the obesity epidemic more generally. Numerous popular press articles reporting on medical studies, medical studies themselves, and the Centers for Disease Control and Prevention all equate fat bodies with higher risk of heart disease, stroke, type 2 diabetes, cancer, gallbladder disease, sleep apnea, respiratory problems, and bone and joint degeneration. As a result, it's not surprising that many of the people featured on medicalized programs share with viewers at home, through both stories and visual displays amenable to the audience being able to conduct an at-home diagnosis of the bodies on the screen, the ways in which their bodies are diseased because of their experiences of fatness. For instance, Henry (season 1, episode 3) suffers from high blood pressure, sleep apnea, and the inability to walk, all physical impairments or conditions commonly related to the disease of obesity. Similarly, Donald (season 1, episode 2) suffers from severe cellulitis (a painful and persistent bacterial infection of the skin), which he attributes to both his skin being stretched due to his large size and water retention caused by his physical immobility.

On *Cherry Healey: Old Before My Time* (2013), Claire takes thirty pills a day to manage her "obesity-related diseases," which include depression, acid reflux, and gout. *Old Before My Time*'s narrator adds that Claire could also suffer from arthritis, intestinal problems, cancer, diabetes, liver disease, high blood pressure, blocked arteries, stroke, and low self-esteem if she does not lose weight. The doctor treating her in the episode further explains that Claire's life span would decrease by fifteen years if any of these "obesity-related diseases" does develop. Likewise, on *Fat Doctor* (2007–2012), Dr. Slater says of Jean that her weight puts her at risk of diabetes, high blood pressure, and heart disease, adding that she "will inevitably die young." The show's narrator then dramatically reinforces the message: "Unless she loses weight soon, she will be dead in the next five years." On the *Body Shock* episode "Half Ton Son" (2009), Billy's doctor's medical assessment is that his weight is overtaxing his heart and lungs, reducing his life expectancy to no more than a couple of years. The only solution, according to doctors on the series, is to reduce the amount of fat on his body through gastric bypass surgery, but the surgery cannot be performed because Billy's fat layer prevents doctors from reaching his stomach laparoscopically. Therefore, the doctor opts to perform a "tummy tuck" and remove sixty-nine pounds of healthy tissue in the form of abdominal fat in order to eventually complete the gastric bypass surgery and several additional skin removal surgeries. Many of the participants on these shows do not yet have—and maybe never will have—most of the "obesity-related diseases" discussed by doctors, but their bodies are already seen as diseased because they are fat and thus automatically considered at risk for disease.

These "obesity-related diseases" plus the physical impairment, social disability, and feelings of being "near death" experienced by participants inevitably lead to the "treating" of fat on one's body through weight-loss surgery. As Ashley says, "Diet and exercise alone is not going to help the situation that I'm in. I need the medical intervention." Generally, for those categorized as "dangerously obese," like the participants on *My 600-lb Life* and similar TV programs, medical treatment become the "only" way for people to "overcome" their diseased or physically impaired bodies, even though "success" rates are low. The show reiterates this through screen text, such as, "In a last ditch effort to change her life, Penny hopes to get weight-loss surgery," and narrative explanations like those in the second season opening credits: "If I could do it without surgery, I would have done it." Melissa also views gastric bypass surgery as the only barrier standing between her and death: "I can either die on the operating table because I'm trying to get healthy, or I can die because I'm six hundred pounds. At least I tried."

Other series echo this same message of surgery being the only option. The narrator of *Fat Doctor* describing Sasha evidences this: "Diets have failed and weight-loss surgery was the only option left." Sasha then echoes a similar sentiment herself, saying, "I don't have a choice. If I don't have it I'm going to die." Similarly, the narrator for the "Half Ton Man" (2006) episode of *Body Shock* says of its participant, Patrick, "There is now only one way to stop him from eating: gastric bypass surgery." On *The Man Who Ate Himself to Death* (2013), Ricky, who has not been able to leave his house for seven years, dies before he is able to undergo weight-loss surgery, supporting a bariatric surgeon on the show's claim, "If he doesn't get help he will die. For patients that are super obese the best option for weight-loss is surgery."

Anticipating criticism over the reliance on surgery and the notion that bariatric surgery is a form of cheating in order to achieve an idealized body,[57] which demonstrate the dominance of the obesity epidemic health discourse connecting fatness to a lack of self-control or self-discipline, Dr. Shaw of *Fat Doctor* explains, "People say 'obesity is self-created and that people should lose weight by themselves,' but this indicates a complete failure of understanding the prejudice that these people feel. They have tried everything else and if you call their chance at life 'cheating,' then you are missing the point." One individual on Australia's *Big: Extreme Makeover* is worried about her upcoming surgery, but decides it's worth it, saying, "For me it's a win-win. If I come out of the surgery, my children are free. If I die in the surgery, my children are free." These medical programs frequently discuss death as a potential result of fatness; individuals *may* die because of their surgeries, but they *will* die (according to the television doctors) if they do not have them.

Not only is surgery positioned as the only option for reducing the amount of fat on "super morbidly obese" bodies, but the simple act of fat removal is also equated with getting healthier even if nothing else about the patient's health status changes. For example, just before Henry undergoes his surgery, Dr. Nowzaradan asks him, "Are you ready to get healthier?," implying that the removal of skin and fatty tissue is the route to health, as opposed to considering his health status holistically by dealing with emotional and psychological issues that may lead to overeating or mitigating his problematic home context, which the show describes as full of "food-enablers."

By this point each episode begins to vary significantly, as individual experiences deviate much like the weight-loss narratives discussed in chapter 5. Instead of the common narrative sequence of exhibiting the fat body as a spectacle to foster shame, changing the body through weight loss, and revealing the "new" body, potential transformation on *My 600-lb Life* is far more contingent and fraught with problems as most participants falter, treatments fail, and Dr. Now-zaradan is unable to alleviate bodily problems like so many miraculous TV doctors before him. After meeting with Dr. Nowzaradan, participants are required to "prove" they can manage or change their relationships with food by losing a set amount of weight prior to being approved for weight-loss surgery. This is a somewhat perplexing situation since virtually all participants previously express the difficulty or impossibility of losing weight on their own, but the desire to qualify for surgery to change or save their life seems to operate as a more powerful motivator than previous experiences, diagnoses, risks, and experiences of shame or humiliation. Most participants are put on diets limiting their food intake from five hundred to twelve hundred calories a day and need to lose between thirty and one hundred pounds before surgery. Some participants, such as Ashley (season 5, episode 2), are able to achieve this easily, which raises the question, if Ashley is able to lose weight through diet and exercise, why is that "treatment" not continued long term? Why does Dr. Nowzaradan recommend an invasive and high-risk surgery that does not have particularly good long-term health outcomes? Other participants have a much more difficult time losing weight prior to surgery, with some taking months to lose the requisite amount, especially participants Penny and Charity. In fact, both Penny and Charity struggle to lose weight even while hospitalized and on a strictly controlled diet. Furthermore, both struggle to lose weight after surgery, with both being intermittently hospitalized and neither making "good progress," according to Dr. Nowzaradan, toward achieving their weight-loss goals.

This lack of progress toward weight loss goals while under constant surveillance also happens on *Inside Brookhaven Obesity Clinic*. One participant, Vince, who returns to Brookhaven—an inpatient medical weight-loss facility—after gaining weight postrelease, resists many of the clinic's rules and orders fast food to be delivered to his hospital room. Commenting on the situation, one of the clinic's doctors tells the camera crew, "We can't just say 'no food in the building.' To treat an addiction we have to modify their behavior and change their lifestyles to see results. We can't lock everybody up." Yet their attempts to change Vince's behavior, evidenced by him being admitted twice to Brookhaven, do not seem to be working either.

The "failures" of Penny, Charity, and Vince to lose weight despite being hospitalized and undergoing surgery are interesting for several reasons. First, both of those forms of medical treatment are framed as the "only" options, yet even these options prove not to be particularly successful at controlling or treating the body. Second, as Weber argues in her analysis of makeover programs, participants who are resistant or disobedient are portrayed as difficult, and "failure to comply is punished by shaming,"[58] which is also generally the case in *My 600-lb Life*. But because the series frames these attempts of bodily transformation as necessary for treating disease—as no longer being a choice but rather a requirement

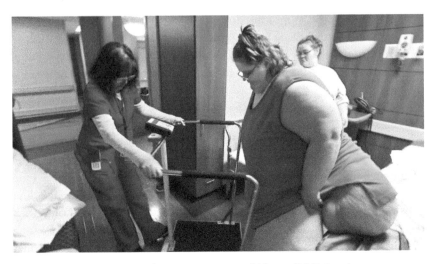

Figure 12   Charity on season 3 of *My 600-lb Life* (2015)

for living—this situation is framed as more dire, coupling shame with sympathy and compassion. In both cases Dr. Nowzaradan acknowledges the limitations of surgical treatment and hospitalization without getting to the "root cause" of why each participant overeats through therapy (why therapy is not recommended as a first step in treatment is unknown, but it would likely diminish the narrative tensions created by the show), which creates a more complex understanding of fat embodiment, as well as weight gain and weight loss, typically found on weight-loss reality television.

Third, when Penny, Charity, and Vince resist treatments within the hospital, it challenges that space as a site where discipline is easily exerted over the body. On *My 600-lb Life*, not only is the constant surveillance of the television camera not enough to "control" Penny, Charity, and other participants through their yearlong journeys (and in follow-up episodes years later), but a primary site of disciplinary power—the hospital—also "fails" in that role. These examples of the insufficiency of constant surveillance, whether in the hospital or via the television, operate much differently than other programs focusing on fatness, which according to Palmer in his analysis of "large bodies" on reality weight-loss shows tend to "offer proof that an increase in surveillance is effective in that nearly everyone loses weight and becomes happier in the process."[59] Like the shows discussed in chapter 5, not only do medicalized fat television programs contradict this "proof," but the described seriousness of each situation coupled with the lack of medical relief again works to foster sympathy as much as shame for the TV participants perceived as embodying the disease of obesity.

As briefly mentioned throughout this chapter, narratives of "food addiction" frequently come up on *My 600-lb Life*, and other series like *Happily Ever After*

(2013), which features a man receiving surgery at one thousand pounds, *Big Medicine* (2007–2015), and *The Real Skinny* (2007) all talk about weight-loss surgery (and later skin removal surgery) in relation to food addiction. One study exploring the addictive potential of food finds that overeating alters and rewards the brain in ways comparable to the repeated use of illicit drugs like cocaine.[60] Numerous television programs reflect and reinforce this notion, evidenced both by the narrator of *Addicted to Food* (2011) describing the "patients" in the first episode as needing to detox from food and "patients" themselves explaining that they compulsively eat and rely on food for comfort and satisfaction. On a season 3 episode of *Fat Doctor*, the narrator says to viewers, "A quarter of British adults are dangerously overweight. For many, however hard they try, they simply cannot control their addiction to food." On the "Half Ton Man" episode of *Body Shock,* one doctor even references a common alcohol addiction idiom when discussing his patient, Rosalie: "I guarantee before she dies she will fall off the wagon." He then goes on to discuss brain similarities between obese individuals and those with drug addictions, explaining that overeating may produce similar responses in the brain as taking illicit drugs. "Overeating becomes addictive. It decreases their dopamine receptors requiring them to eat larger amounts of food to find pleasure." Similarly, on *The Man Who Ate Himself to Death*, one bariatric surgeon compares obesity to alcoholism in the sense that "you're never cured." Although fatness as the "result" of a food addiction clearly complicates health frames of self-discipline and self-control, addiction also reinforces the necessity of treatment under medical authority in helping individuals gain control over the foods they eat.

Where Are They Now? Limitations to Televised
Medical Authority and Treatments

Weight-loss surgeries are consistently framed as the only option for "super morbidly obese" individuals (and overweight individuals, per Dr. Oz) because previous attempts at dieting or exercising have proved unsuccessful. However, despite gastric bypass surgery being framed as the only solution to treat obesity and its causing of physical impairment across most medicalized TV series, the narratives often reveal that solution to be as problematic and flawed as any other weight-loss treatment or intervention. As *My 600-lb Life* fully demonstrates, the solution is not "magic."[61] Even if reducing the size of the stomach diminishes physical hunger pangs, many of the individuals featured on *My 600-lb Life* regain lost weight over time, reflecting the non-TV experiences of those who undergo weight-loss surgery.[62] This is particularly evident on *My 600-lb Life: Where Are They Now?*, where most of the participants describe weight gain, including Melissa (gaining back over one hundred pounds) and Ashley (gaining sixty pounds over just a couple months), or complications resulting in stalled weight loss, particularly

Pauline, who suffers from frequent skin infections and begins gaining weight just one year after surgery. These experiences after weight-loss surgery further reflect nontelevised experiences in that many individuals on- and off-screen experience serious side effects as a result of their surgeries, including decreased metabolic syndrome, weakness, acid reflux, and even fatal malnutrition.[63] Therefore, the treatment for making potentially unhealthy or diseased bodies "healthy" is actually quite risky and potentially detrimental itself and could contribute to other kinds of disease or experiences of physical impairment.[64]

Furthermore, weight-loss surgery does not address the underlying motivation to overeat. For example, Tara finds her behavior postsurgery to be similar to her behavior presurgery. Even though Dr. Nowzaradan says prior to her surgery that it is the only option, he explains to the camera, "Tara is overeating and not being truthful about it. . . . If the patient doesn't want to change they will convince themselves they are not eating very much." When Tara tells her side of the story after meeting with Dr. Nowzaradan, she says, "I can't change overnight. Changing something like my eating habits is not easy because I'm doing what I know. I may cheat here or there, but I am trying." The continued impulse to eat presents a serious challenge to the efficacy of weight-loss surgery as a medical treatment under medical authority, or at least to weight-loss surgery as an "only" option considering the fact that its success depends on multiple treatments addressing everything from the physical to the emotional. Reflecting these issues, most follow-up episodes for *My 600-lb Life* portray a majority of individuals either gaining weight back or no longer losing, while deemed by medical authorities to still be obese postsurgery. Most follow-up news articles about participants similarly detail the difficulties of sustaining or continuing weight-loss postsurgery.[65] Yet individuals are still encouraged to risk their lives to undergo weight-loss surgery despite these limited television results, which, again, align with the limited and problematic results of bariatric surgeries more generally. Regardless, the reliance on surgery is a common representation of those medically categorized as super obese because health choices may already have "proven" to be ineffective for weight loss. Medical treatments like bariatric surgeries become both the "last hope" for weight loss and, for some, the "beginning of a terrible mistake."[66]

Notably, neither *My 600-lb Life* nor other medicalized fat TV programs end in the same kind of dramatic transformation from fat to thin that weight-loss programs emphasizing diet and exercise more often do. Therefore, participants are not depicted as "basking in a visuality she or he once avoided"[67] and never reach "after-body" status, which is a departure from transformational reality television and numerous weight-loss programs. This is also a departure from other types of medical-themed television where a majority of the exhibited medical procedures will have a positive outcome or are "dominated by the trajectory form ill-health to cure."[68] In fact, success, in terms of reducing the amount of adipose tissue to be within the "healthy" BMI weight range, is rarely achieved by any medicalized fat TV participants regardless of medical treatment or submission to medical authority. Further, and as previously discussed, several participants experience negative outcomes postsurgery, with one participant, Dominique, passing away just two weeks after surgery (as documented on the 2012 TLC special *600 Pound Mom: A Race Against Time*).

However, despite the lack of "success" in achieving weight loss through medical alternatives to diet and exercise, these medicalized shows do work to reinforce the notion that fat individuals still have an obligation, not to typical dieting or exercising regimens, perhaps, but to following the treatments outlined by medical authorities. Just like health-oriented weight-loss TV programs, then, medicalized programs are still, largely, characterized by neoliberal discourses that "incite good citizens to take care of their own health; they punish those who fail to live up to this socially constructed moral obligation."[69] These reality TV healers are not always able to treat their patients' bodies, negotiating the way medical doctors have long been portrayed on television and fostering greater sympathy for the participants on these shows. Of course there is always the potential that these situations can be read as the fault of the participant or patient, too, as we cannot fully escape the omnipresent umbrella of personal responsibility within the neoliberal era.

Conclusion

Medicalized fat television programs reinforce the notion that fatness is a disease of obesity, something that needs to be treated rather than a state of being that can either be "overcome" through diet and exercise or accepted as just another way to be in the world. However, *My 600-lb Life* falls short of persuading viewers of the value of currently used obesity treatments like bariatric surgery and hospitalization. Just like weight-loss television focusing on exercise and calorie restriction in the vein of health discourses, medicalized understandings of fatness are inadvertently debated more than they are straightforwardly reinforced. Thus, representations on medicalized fat television texts act as important sites for exploring negotiations between medical authority and individual agency over the body; they strengthen medical authority and legitimize the necessity of medical treatments for fatness, but also concurrently challenge hierarchical power over the body and the efficacy of surgery and hospitalization. The negotiation of these issues, labeling of fatness as a disease, and the spectacular portrayals of the fat body position participants on the show in more sympathetic ways; they are unable to help themselves and medical authorities are unable to fully and truly help them too. Furthermore, the reliance on these types of medicalized treatments for fatness and the positioning of health practices, like diet and exercise, as being necessary but ultimately insufficient for weight loss poke holes in the dominant logics of the obesity epidemic and its emphasis on personal responsibility and individualism.

Medicalized shows thus put forth an alternative way of thinking about fatness, and alternative "solutions" for reducing the amount of fat on one's body, but like their more dominant television counterparts, medicalized fat television programs ultimately fail to demonstrate the viability of those alternative "solutions" for long-term or significant weight loss. In fact, despite surgery or hospitalization being the "last" chance or "only" option for TV participants, there is an even smaller potential of achieving the (illusory) "after-body."

The failures and inconsistencies present across all these medicalized texts also undermine television's ability to govern at a distance. While inadvertently showing that medical authority over the body and medical treatments like surgery, hospitalization, and pharmaceutical therapy are ineffective, inconsistent, or problematic for other reasons, these shows also demonstrate that being under constant surveillance of the television camera does not help in achieving weight loss or transformation. These TV programs may extend the reach of medical authority and traditional sites for disciplining the body throughout our society of control, yet at the same time both medical authority over the body and television's ability to discipline our bodies at a distance are negotiated.

7

Celebrating Large Bodies
on the Small Screen

FROM FAT VISIBILITY TO
FAT POSITIVITY

After two date requests and the gifting of expensive hockey tickets, Vanessa, a new waitress at the Comedy Cellar on FX's *Louie* (2010–2015), finally gets Louie to agree to an afternoon coffee date. Their envy-inspiring great first date includes a stroll through the city while sharing stories and telling jokes, that is until Louie absent-mindedly quips about the difficulty of dating in New York City. Also sensitive to the issue of dating in the city, Vanessa retorts, "Try dating in your late thirties as a fat girl!" Through a lengthy monologue, Vanessa explains how much it "sucks" to be a fat woman because gendered expectations for beauty and desirability construct a double standard unfair to women. Vanessa goes on to explain that her situation sucks even more because fat women are not supposed to talk about how much it sucks to be fat women as it's "too much for people to handle."

Critical reception of this scene varied between praise and apprehension. It's applauded for discussing fat womanhood, even if from the perspective of a man, because the topic is discussed so infrequently throughout television's history.[1] One critic points out Vanessa's monologue positions neither fat itself as a problem nor Vanessa as disliking her fat body, instead identifying the problem as societal; fat individuals and those who associate with them are stigmatized, and fat women are viewed as less than or not good enough, especially by men whose fragile egos rely on having an ideally attractive partner.[2] However, another cultural critic pushed back against all the praise bestowed upon Louis C.K., instead finding the monologue to be condescending to Vanessa because someone as outgoing, smart, and self-assured as she is should expect and demand more than just wanting to hold hands with a "nice guy."[3]

Louie is not the only TV show to consider what it is like to be a fat woman in a society that privileges, and even demands, thinness, although this episode of *Louie* does so with less physical violence and paternalistically protective impulses than other recent television examples. For instance, a 2014 episode of *Homeland* (2011–) depicts CIA operative Quinn drunkenly sleeping with a fat woman while grieving the loss of a colleague. When Quinn and his overnight companion go out for breakfast the following morning, a group of men a few tables over share fat jokes and laugh at the size of the woman's body (she does not have a name in the episode, a problem in itself). Angered by their behavior (and channeling a significant amount of aggression), Quinn confronts the men, breaking the hand of one and bloodying the face of another. Likewise, although airing several years earlier than *Homeland* and *Louie*, John Sacrimoni of *The Sopranos* (1999–2007) defends his wife, Ginnie, after members of Tony Soprano's mafia family joke about Ginnie being so large as to need a ninety-pound mole removed from her backside. John assaults and urinates on one of the offenders, justifying his actions as being in defense of his wife's honor. Later he explains to Tony that women experience fatness differently and with more difficultly than men do, although he considers Ginnie to be beautiful and "Rubenesque."

These television examples explore a kind of duality of fatness, reinforcing the notion that fat is undesirable, or perceived as undesirable by many (although clearly desirable by the characters in these episodes), yet nevertheless a type of body that should be understood with compassion and kindness like every other type of body. After all, the individuals harassing, joking about, or devaluing fat women are positioned as far more of a problem than fat embodiment itself. Although none of these series can really be categorized as body positive or fat accepting, nor do any of them necessarily strive to be, these particular episodes do give visibility to fat women, albeit briefly, and bear witness to the insensitive and unkind interpersonal interactions many fat individuals experience on a daily basis.

These particular scenes and episodes exploring fatness are part of a growing number of TV programs representing a greater diversity of body types, including *Drop Dead Diva* (2009–2014), *Huge* (2010), *Super Fun Night* (2013–2014), *Mike & Molly* (2010–2016), *Big Sexy* (2011), *Curvy Girls* (2011–2013), *Fat Friends* (2000–2005), *My Mad Fat Diary* (2013–2015), *Ruby* (2008–2011), *More to Love* (2009), *My Big Fat Fabulous Life* (2015–), and *Big Women, Big Love* (2015). These programs not only depict a diversity of body types across the small screen but also generally promote body positivity and the acceptance—and even celebration—of the many shapes and sizes that bodies can be as opposed to framing fat bodies as objects for shaming and discipline, or intervention and treatment.

Many of these television programs also counter fat stereotypes and health and medical discourses of fatness positioning fat individuals as unhappy, unhealthy, or unable to actually live their lives until they lose weight. Moreover, these shows embrace a sensitivity to fatness not found on health-influenced weight-loss programs or medicalized texts that frame fat bodies as diseased and in need of treatment. Discussing the positive impact on body image in relation to fatness on *Mike & Molly*, Melissa McCarthy says, "Any time you see a broad spectrum of people on TV, it's good. It's good to have something a little more realistic, so people aren't always striving to be these unrealistic role models and then giving up. 'Oh, I could never be that perfect.' Well, guess what? No one is, except on this tiny little studio set somewhere in Hollywood. I think a show like *Mike & Molly* takes the pressure off of some people. Subconsciously, it may make people take it a little easier on themselves."[4] However, fat TV programs embracing body size diversity through fat visibility, body positivity, or fat positivity are not always well received because of the dominance (and "common sense" status) of health and medicalized discourses of fatness in the context of the obesity epidemic. So even though an individual developing a positive body image is widely accepted as important for emotional and physical well-being, the same logics are not consistently extended to fat individuals, especially fat women. For example, a 2013 op-ed for the *Boston Globe* exemplifies the tension between body positivity and the perceived necessity of excluding those whose body positivity includes fat acceptance because it is viewed as promoting obesity: "Unrealistic ideals of bodily perfection certainly exist, and cause many, especially women and girls, to harm themselves through fad diets or obsessive exercise. The message that beauty and health come in different shapes and sizes is a positive one in moderation. But fat acceptance is no improvement on the thinness cult."[5] This less than inclusive notion of body positivity actually helps explain the emergence and growing influence of explicit fat acceptance, which rejects constructions of the obesity epidemic, automatic assumptions positioning fat as inherently unhealthy, the ways in which fat bodies are medicalized in relation to disease, and how body positivity itself isn't always extended to fat women. Yet fatness remains articulated to these ideas and, if not understood in relation to them, then in defense of them.

Fat-positive TV, which reflects discourses of fat acceptance, as well as television shows depicting body size diversity and foregrounding messages of body positivity bridge the gap between the idealized, unrealistically thin bodies most often found throughout television's history and the super morbidly obese bodies found in the medicalized fat television programs discussed in chapter 6. The fat bodies and fat TV discussed in this chapter are positioned not as funny like Jackie Gleason's character was on *The Honeymooners* (1955–1956) or scary like Alfred Hitchcock's robust and eerie silhouette on *Alfred Hitchcock Presents* (1955–1962), but rather as human, as like the bodies we see every day or like our own bodies. This chapter, then, explores representations across multiple series of fatness or non–normatively idealized bodies reflecting discourses oppositional to or copresent with those found in chapters 5 and 6. In other words, these fat representations range from existing alongside to directly challenging discourses of health in connection to the obesity epidemic and the medicalization of fat bodies. These shows reflect body-positive and fat-acceptance discourses focusing less on *the body* of a character or participant, and more on the *whole person*, a person who may just happen to be fat. Camryn Manheim's character Ellenor Frutt on *The Practice* (1997–2004) is an example of this kind of body size diversity. Though fatness was never discussed on the show, Mannheim gleefully shouted in her Emmy acceptance speech for the role, "I gladly carry the torch for big women. This is for all the fat girls!"[6]

In addition to the sporadic body size diversity found on shows like *The Practice*, some programs intermittently address fatness across different scenes or episodes, such as *Drop Dead Diva* and *Mike & Molly*, while others commit to consistently reinforcing particular kinds of body and fat positivity, like *Big Sexy*, *Curvy Girls*, and *Huge*. TV shows articulated to discourses of body positivity and fat acceptance are increasingly present; however, they more often demonstrate the social politics and attitudes of individual actors, creators, producers, and network executives within the television industry rather than already established industry lore. But as many of these shows prove relatable to large audiences and are successful across broadcast networks as well as cable and streaming channels, demonstrating their potential for profitability and resonance among young, socially conscious viewers, we will likely see more of them. For instance, eight million people consistently watched CBS's *Mike &d Molly*, a large enough viewership in the post-network era to make it the number one show on its night and in its time slot. Similarly, TLC's *My Big Fat Fabulous Life* ranks number one in its Tuesday night slot, lifting TLC up to number two in overall viewers for the night. As the television industry notes the success of these programs, emergent industry lore begins to form and circulate throughout niche media outlets, including on blogs, on "Insta-lebrity" accounts, and across advertising campaigns, and may eventually become more prominent among television executives.

According to Timothy Havens, industry lore, or the organizational common sense of media industries, "marks the boundaries of how industry insiders imagine television programming, its audiences, and the kinds of textual practices that can and cannot be profitable."[7] But industry lore is not necessarily homogenous or static; instead, Havens contends technological as well as economic and global market changes, as well as social and cultural changes, prompt new forms of industry lore to develop. This emerging industry lore then leads to new practices and even particular kinds of representations.[8] This chapter thus details one example of how industry lore emerges, or to use Havens's phrase, how lore "bubbles up from below,"[9] as alternative ways of thinking and resistant social politics held by individual actors, creators, producers, and executives within the television industry make their way to the screen. In fact, television has a long history of balancing the social politics of individual actors, such as support for feminism on *Cagney and Lacy* (1981–1988) and civil rights on *Soul Train* (1971–2006), with existing audience assumptions and industry practices, which ultimately contributes to developing lore and representational shifts over time.[10]

This chapter examines the emerging relationship between bodies/fatness and media industries, and discusses trends across fat TV programs, including programs representing body diversity and/or circulating messages of body positivity and fat positivity. While body-positive programs are increasingly common, contributing to emerging industry lore, fat-acceptance or fat-positive programs remain rare as they directly counter dominant discourses of the obesity epidemic, making them somewhat controversial and perhaps more financially precarious for TV producers and channels. Moreover, this is the first chapter including scripted programming in its analysis, although the lines between scripted and reality programs, which are also typically scripted to various degrees, continue to blur. For the purposes of this chapter, I treat scripted and "nonscripted" television programs in the same manner, as I am most interested in the similarities found across narratives and representations rather than teasing out how the marker of "reality" may influence the way the text is read by viewers. Finally, this chapter is most focused on representations within the United States and on representations of women. Fat men are more commonly depicted on television and have been throughout television's history (as I discussed in chapter 1), but the bodies of fat men are almost never represented in relation to body positivity or fat acceptance, except when they are interested in body-positive and fat-accepting women. This trend is likely the result of the fat-acceptance and body-positivity movements primarily being composed of women and deeply connected to feminism in their resistance to the body-aesthetic demands perpetuated by patriarchal society. And, of course, these movements and instances of resistance are the result of fat prejudice and fat stigmatization disproportionately and detrimentally affecting women in numerous ways.[11]

Emerging Industry Lore

Connected to the selling of particular products is the selling of particular body-positive fat TV programs. In fact, there is growing discussion about the need for, impetus behind, and relatability of body diversity on television, which deviates from typical industry lore regarding the depiction of fat individuals. David Ehlers, director of ZenithOptimedia, argues that even early shows about weight loss, such as *The Biggest Loser*, ran contrary to industry logics: "I had people say that fat people weren't attractive and that nobody wants to see fat people on television. I said, 'Well, do you know anyone who is fat?' 'Oh yea,' they said, 'my mother is, my sister and brother is.' So, I told them that if everyone in this room knows someone who's in that situation, isn't that your audience?"[12] The overall success and high ratings of something like *The Biggest Loser*, then, according to its own production president, Chad Bennett, helped tear down walls to fat representation.[13] Rita Mullin, the program development vice president of TLC, which airs a large number of fat television programs, speaks about this change in logic and the way it has evolved since the early 2000s: "You can't ignore how successful 'The Biggest Loser' has been, but more than that, society is looking at the issue in a different way now. The kind of programming we're doing on cable reflects that. We're putting a human face to what had been, before, a punchline. When you watch a show like *650-Pound Virgin* or *Ruby* suddenly you realize, 'I can identify with this person.'"[14] Similarly, Sally Ann Salsano, who produced both *Dance Your Ass Off* and *More to Love*, talks about her own identification with the people featured on her programs: "I'm overweight, and I'm not going to do a show that makes fun of fat people, because I know what that feels like. I have a connection with my cast on these shows." These shows are also viewed as friendly to a number of advertisers, including Lane Bryant, a plus-size clothing store for women, which helps produce Fox's *More to Love*.[15]

There is a growing sense among television critics and individuals working in the industry that "if there is one thing that fat people hate seeing on television, it's shows where large people get screamed at to lose weight."[16] And given the large number of people categorized or self-identifying as fat, there is a potentially huge audience for content friendly to fatness. In fact, Fox executive Mike Darnell argues there no longer needs to be the "axiom that people need to be ultra thin or ultra good-looking on TV," instead insisting that network executives and producers are working to create shows considered "inspirational in nature" instead of exploitative of fat individuals. Michael Schneider, who is a writer for *Variety*, also says, "With so many TV viewers struggling with their weight, showcasing more realistically-sized people on reality TV would seem to be a no-brainer."[17] These assumptions about what will appeal to audiences are also intertwined with both industry and critical discussions of the potential impact of these shifts in storytelling and representations. It's argued that fat visibility on TV could reduce social biases against fat individuals,[18] while representations sensitive to fat stigma could correct "reflexive cultural judgments levied against the overweight at a time when obesity has been cast as one of the greatest blights of our age."[19]

Televising Body Positivity

As body size diversity on the small screen continues to translate to critical acclaim and/or high ratings, emergent industry lore adds to and amends the dominant logics circulated within media industries. So, in addition to body size diversity through greater fat visibility, there are also television programs more explicitly, albeit still intermittently, engaging in body-positive storylines. For instance, Fox and now Hulu's *The Mindy Project* (2012–2017) receives a significant amount of critical praise, and it reached three to four million viewers per episode its first two seasons, ranking in the top ten among women in the "eighteen to thirty-four-year-old women" demographic. In early episodes of *The Mindy Project*, Mindy explains, "Do you know how hard it is for a chubby thirty-one-year-old woman to go on a legit date with a guy who majored in economics at Duke?" Mindy Kaling, the main character, writer, and creative force behind *The Mindy Project*, later explains in an interview why she incorporates discussions of weight on the show: "I wanted to write a female character who's strong enough that a man's criticizing her weight or looks can sting but not devastate her. Too many women give others too much power over their self-worth."[20] Sheila Moeschen for the *Huffington Post* praises Kaling's body positivity: "By refusing to make body criticism a focal point of the show (in terms of plot and character development), Kaling embraces the notion that more women could benefit from spending less time preoccupied with body transformation and more time enjoying and accepting themselves."[21] Yet some episodes of *The Mindy Project* demonstrate Mindy's preoccupation with the appearance and size of her body. In a second season episode, "Danny C Is My Personal Trainer," Mindy panics when her boyfriend, Danny, wants to take her on a romantic vacation because it necessitates wearing a bikini in front of him (he has yet to see her naked, and she hides her body from all of her sexual partners). To get her body "bikini ready," Mindy spends a majority of the episode exercising with Danny as her coach. But soon she becomes frustrated with his personal training style, saying to him, "Just because you have like zero percent body fat and eat only three meals a day and never snack doesn't mean you can tell me what's wrong with my body." However, after rejecting the body criticism of others, Mindy herself goes on to list all of her perceived faults, including her "fat knees" and cellulite, but Danny disagrees: "I know you are self-conscious but you don't need to be. . . . You are a woman and that's good. Look like a woman." This episode reflects theories about how differences that normatively mark bodies as female, such as having large hips, stomachs, breasts, and thighs, ironically become "most of the ways in which women feel physically 'wrong.'"[22] The takeaway message from this episode of *The Mindy Project* is clearly one of body positivity, albeit through external validation rather than internal self-acceptance or self-celebration. Mindy ultimately struggles with her body image and size acceptance, as many women do, vacillating between insecurity and confidence.

The television series *Girls* (2012–2017) functions similarly to *The Mindy Project*. Although *Girls* was lucky to reach one million viewers per episode, its presence on HBO automatically provides it with cultural cache and buzz in the popular press, and as a result it received numerous industry awards, including an Emmy, Golden Globe, and Writer's Guild Award. Hannah, the main character played by Lena Dunham, doesn't regularly talk about her body beyond saying in the final episode of season 1, "I am thirteen pounds overweight and it has been awful for me my whole life," but she frequently puts her non–aesthetically idealized body on display. Numerous scenes depict Hannah in the nude, including her eating a cupcake in a bathtub, disrobing before having sex, wearing a see-through mesh tank top during a coke-fueled night of partying, donning a green bikini for the duration of an entire episode, and playing a naked game of ping-pong. Hannah fearlessly and nonchalantly exhibits her naked body, and by doing so she rejects the "rules" of "acceptable" behavior by someone who believes she is carrying more weight than she should.

Reviews of both *The Mindy Project* and *Girls* generally praise Kaling and Dunham for their body positivity and what they "get right" about body image,[23] although *Girls* also receives a significant amount of criticism. For instance, Joan Rivers criticized Dunham for her frequent nudity on *Girls*, saying, "You are sending a message out to people saying, 'It's okay! Stay fat! Get diabetes. Everybody die! Lose your fingers.'"[24] This kind of reaction is regularly levied against those who advocate fat acceptance, but it's less frequently applied to those who are, according to Dunham's character Hannah, "thirteen pounds overweight." Another reviewer of *Girls* argues that instead of promoting body positivity, Hannah reinforces stereotypes of fatness as she eats a lot, specifically referencing her eating a cupcake while soaking in the bathtub, and "does not seem to care about her appearance." The reviewer further suggests Dunham uses her body both for laughs and as an "extension of all the things wrong with her . . . as a measure of personal failing."[25] In contrast, I do not interpret Hannah as using her body for laughs, not that such a thing would be inherently problematic, and instead interpret her as resisting and playing with norms of beauty and style rather than being oblivious to them. In fact, the reviewer's assumption that Hannah does not care about her appearance or body size relies on accepting aesthetic idealizations and health norms as the standard from which Hannah deviates, whether purposefully or obliviously.

Similarly and predictably, Dunham's character, Hannah, frequently garners comparison to Kaling's character, Mindy. For example, another reviewer critiques Hannah for "not giving a hoot about what others think of her looks," which she considers to be unrealistic, whereas Mindy "totally cares how she looks," which instead offers viewers "a model of a woman who likes to look good, and wouldn't mind losing a little weight, but doesn't base her self-worth on it."[26] Instead of arguing that one representation is "better" than the other, both kinds of body size diversity are important. Neither example is a "right" way or a "wrong" way of being body positive; rather, these two series in conjunction with other fat- and body-positive TV programs (as well as zines, Instagram posts, and Tumblrs) depict various body experiences as well as intrapersonal relationships with the body. While Hannah is perhaps more radical in her body positivity, particularly in terms of embracing the size and shape of her body through frequent nudity, Mindy is possibly more relatable to a wider range of viewers—viewers who are more likely to also idealize thinness, but be against body shaming. More important than which show is more body positive than the other is whether each show's messages of body positivity extend to those beyond a size ten. It remains to be seen how viewers might respond to a three- or four-hundred-pound woman embracing her nudity on the small screen because it has yet to actually happen.

Televising Fat Positivity and Fat Acceptance

Although Mindy Kaling and Lena Dunham actively contribute to television's body size diversity, both actresses and their characters are fairly normative in size—neither would be categorized as plus size per fashion industry standards, and both are unlikely to experience the same kinds or same levels of stigmatization, discrimination, and social judgment many fat individuals report experiencing. However, there are a small number of TV shows representing fat, nonidealized bodies without focusing on weight loss. Although weight or goals of weight loss may provide a foundational premise for some television series, it is rarely a sustained narrative focus on programs like *Drop Dead Diva, Huge,* and *Mike & Molly*. To varying degrees across these programs, weight is a nonissue, a "small" issue, or an issue discussed with more complexity than simple recommendations and expressed desires to lose weight. In an interview with *Ad Age,* a spokesperson for Lifetime refers to *Drop Dead Diva* as a "mainstream show that happens to have a plus-size character in the lead role." Peggy Howell, the public relations director for the National Association to Advance Fat Acceptance, offers a statement of support for the lead character, Jane: "Her weight is not an issue. She is not obsessed with dieting. She is living life to its fullest, as are many fat women and men in this country today." ABC Family (now known as Freeform) expresses similar goals in the creation of *Huge*. The network's executive vice-president of advertising sales, Laura Nathanson, says of the show, "*Huge* . . . deals with issues that speak to our millennial audience. Like all of our shows, it deals with topics that are important to young adults, including friendships, parents, rivalries, as well as issues of body image and self-esteem."[27] Even Chuck Lorre, the executive producer of CBS's *Mike & Molly,* offers a similar description of his sitcom: "This isn't a show about weight. It's a show about people trying to make their lives better and find someone that they can have a committed relationship with. If we're still talking about [weight] come episode six, we've got a serious problem, because it would get tired really quickly."[28]

Drop Dead Diva features a fat woman as a successful lawyer. The show debuted in 2009 to almost three million viewers, one of Lifetime's largest audiences for an original scripted series,[29] and continued as one of the channel's most successful shows for its six-season run. Weight is discussed across numerous episodes of *Drop Dead Diva,* but typically in terms of self-acceptance and fat positivity as opposed to weight loss. In fact, the program features a fat main character, Jane, who is professionally and romantically successful, incredibly smart and kind, and uninterested in dieting. Jane is represented as enjoying her life in contrast to narratives found on other fat television texts positioning fat embodiment as an obstacle to overcome for happiness. Across numerous TV programs, losing weight is connected to promises of self-betterment, whether it's becoming a better father (*The Biggest Loser*), finding a girlfriend (*I Used to Be Fat*), overcoming addiction (*Heavy*), becoming pregnant (*The Biggest Loser*), having sex for the first time (*Heavy*), winning a romantic partner back (*Ruby*), or living "happily ever after" (*Shedding for the Wedding*). Instead, *Drop Dead Diva* presents an example of a fat female character who is "comfortable in her own skin" and "unimpeded by not embodying the physically ideal."[30] A TV critic at the *Washington Post* refers to the show as "a refreshing antidote to TV's recent obsession with overweight-themed shows. . . . Instead of pandering to stereotypes, thereby humiliating real people on national television, 'Diva' promotes poignant lessons about body image and society's definition of acceptable beauty."[31]

While the show has many fat-positive moments throughout numerous episodes, its premise is a bit more problematic: a heavenly mix-up results in Deb, who is a thin twentysomething model, returning to earth as Jane, a fat thirtysomething lawyer with an affinity for cats and needlepoint. While Jane was always a confident person, she becomes even more so when Deb begins inhabiting her body. Deb updates Jane's wardrobe, starts wearing makeup, and does a conditioning treatment on her hair. While this series as a whole relays body- and fat-positive messages about beauty coming in many shapes and sizes and encourages us all to be less judgmental of body size, it nevertheless reinforces, at least inadvertently, the idea that there is a thin person trapped inside each fat body.[32] In the case of *Drop Dead Diva*, thin Deb is literally trapped inside fat Jane. But the difference between Deb being trapped in *Drop Dead Diva* and those individuals who feel trapped inside their own fat bodies on *The Biggest Loser* is that Deb as Jane ultimately accepts instead of rejects her body and does not work toward her past thin ideal. Brooke Elliott, who plays Deb/Jane, explains, "We're conditioned to believe that beauty comes in one specific package, but this project is dispelling that myth, saying that beauty is everywhere, in every body type, in every type of person. I was really drawn to this project because of that message and the way it's dealt with in such a fun, but also emotional, way. The most important thing is that we get across to people that you don't have to be a size zero to have worth, to like yourself, or to love your body. As Deb tries to find that, as she tries to accept this new body she's in, that's what keeps me going."[33] While some of Deb's appearance-focused attitude carries over to when she becomes Jane, especially in regard to her bodily presentation, Deb does discontinue her strict dieting routine, terminates her "no eating after seven P.M." rule, and instead begins eating enjoyable foods without guilt. In this way, *Drop Dead Diva* actively counters messages circulated by *The Biggest Loser* and other weight-loss programs, which reinforce the idea that weight loss is primarily about willpower, diet, and exercise. When Deb/Jane's friend Stacy questions why Deb/Jane is not losing weight, considering Deb's previous ability to maintain a very low body weight, Deb/Jane explains to Stacy that while Deb craved grapefruit and celery, Jane's body craves chocolate donuts and sandwiches. Likewise, to maintain her model physique, Deb worked out multiple hours a day, obsessing over every detail of her body, but Deb as Jane discovers she does not have the energy or inclination to exercise after pulling all-nighters at her law firm. According to Josh Berman, creator of *Drop Dead Diva*, these character and narrative decisions explicitly comment on weight in relation to diet and beauty: "I don't believe it's about willpower. If it were, then the assumption would be that if we all wanted to be a size zero, we could be a size zero. Everyone has different needs and desires. If someone finds a doughnut to be comforting, who are we to judge them?"[34]

Drop Dead Diva even engages directly with many issues taken up by fat-acceptance activists; and when doing so, the series focuses less on Jane's body and more on the way thin idealizations and fat stigma affect people more broadly. For instance, one of Jane's clients, Lucy, sues for wrongful termination as she believes she was fired for gaining weight. As the legal narrative unfolds, the series references different sides of the debate over whether fatness should be considered a disability. A few episodes later, Jane takes on the dieting industry for selling "speed disguised as nutritional supplements" to young girls. In another episode, Jane sues a clothing retailer after being poorly treated by a sales associate in a store that does not carry women's plus-size clothing. The associate tells Jane that the dress she admires is intended for a "different silhouette," encouraging her to instead find something "flowy" at another store for "people like her." By episode's end, Jane settles the lawsuit by convincing the store's majority shareholder it would be financially advantageous to carry plus-size clothes, considering the large market of women underserved by the fashion industry and in need of clothing options.

Like *Drop Dead Diva*, ABC Family's *Huge* focuses on body image in relation to self-esteem by promoting body and fat positivity. Although the show lasted only one season, averaging one and a half million viewers per episode, the importance of its body politics outweighs its limited audience. *Huge* stars Nikki Blonsky as Will, a teenager who is happy with her fat body but is nevertheless forced to attend a weight-loss camp (Camp Victory) by her parents. When Will is first weighed in she tells the camp's director, "I know I'm supposed to hate myself, but I don't. I'm okay with the size I am." She echoes a similar sentiment later in the first episode: "Sorry, I'm down with my fat. Me and my fat are like bff. Everyone wants us to hate our bodies and I refuse to." The camp counselor responds by saying, "No one here wants you to hate yourself. We are here for your health." To which Will replies, "Why should I change? Just because my parents are ashamed of how I look? . . . I just think everything you stand for is crap, no offense." Will's resistance to weight loss continues throughout the series. When other campers post magazine photos for "thinspiration," Will posts photos of fat women from the sixteenth century as "fatspiration" while telling everyone her goal is to gain weight at a camp designed for weight loss. To that end, Will even starts an underground junk food trade in protest of being forced to attend Camp Victory.

Of course other campers do desire to lose weight and others still are coded to have disordered eating patterns, but this diversity of fat experiences is precisely what makes *Huge* and its reflections of fat-acceptance discourses so different from the health and medicalized discourses circulated on television. Not all of the campers feel the same way about being fat and not all experience their fatness identically. And like *Drop Dead Diva*, and *Mike & Molly*, which I will discuss shortly, the focus on fatness diminishes as *Huge* progresses, shifting the narrative focus to typical teenage experiences and concerns like sexuality, body odor, difficult parents, friendships, lost journals, and overcoming homesickness. Even though shows like *The Biggest Loser* and *My 600-lb Life* do not solely focus on the body either, as interpersonal drama is just as important as intrapersonal drama for creating narrative interest and tension, *Huge* allows for fat individuals to be well-rounded humans who are fat, but who are not entirely defined by or motivated by being fat.

TV critics also discuss *Huge* and *The Biggest Loser* dichotomously in terms of body messages. Gina Belafonte writes in her 2010 review, "Can Girls Be Overweight and Not Overwrought?" for the *New York Times*, "In this [*Huge*] view fat is a form of social protest, an outcry against the manipulations of a diet-industrial complex. Fringe movements don't often find an arm in the form of hour long dramatic television, but *Huge* . . . stands in some sympathy with a rebellion mounted against so many hours of *The Biggest Loser*."[35] Another review, in *Newsweek*, describes the show as a "heaping helping of 'love your body' instead of fatsploitation," adding, "In an era of Hollywood plastic, Heidi Montag, and *The Biggest Loser*, *Huge* and its curvy stars are immediately refreshing."[36] In fact, one of the creators of *Huge*, Savannah Dooley, says she was immersed in fat-acceptance blogs while writing the show's script, which inspired her to have Will embrace the word "fat" instead of "overweight" because "fat" signifies resistance to normative body discourses reinforcing one standardized, medically prescribed, and aesthetically ideal weight.[37]

Although *Huge* generally embraces discourses of fat acceptance, as well as aspects of health at every size, weight loss is still positioned as important for good health. To that end, ABC Family simultaneously launched the Live Huge campaign, which features recipes created by Jamie Oliver (of ABC's *Jamie Oliver's Food Revolution*) and offers teens advice on how to live healthy lifestyles and improve their self-esteem. Discussing the show and Live Huge, ABC Family executive vice president Kate Juergens explains that while the show is ultimately about self-acceptance, it's also about "coming to terms with taking care of yourself. You want to be the healthiest version of yourself possible, mentally, emotionally, and physically."[38] Implicit in this statement and in the weight-loss-camp backdrop of *Huge* is that weight loss is still tied to being the "healthiest version of yourself," but within the diegetic world of *Huge*, weight loss and loving yourself are not mutually exclusive like they are across weight-loss programs and medicalized texts. These conflicting sentiments, encouraging body and fat positivity and weight loss, are not uncommon across fat-positive texts because of the salience of obesity epidemic rhetoric. Thus, instead of overtly rejecting popularly articulated discourses reflecting public health and medicalized understandings of fatness, which would likely be met with accusations of irresponsibility due to high rates of childhood obesity, in particular *Huge* frames fat positivity and weight loss as copresent and compatible goals instead of oppositional, balancing the physical health of children in accordance with dominant discourses of the obesity epidemic with the mental and emotional health of body and fat positivity in accordance with fat-acceptance discourses.

Even though many of the texts discussed so far are short-lived, reach a small audience, or both, another fat television text, *Mike &d Molly*, proved to have both broad appeal and longevity. *Mike & Molly* features two fat characters who meet at an overeaters anonymous meeting and begin dating. Mike (played by Billy Gardell) is a police officer living by himself in a small apartment and Molly (played by Melissa McCarthy) is a teacher who lives with her mother Joyce and sister Victoria. After the pilot episode's debut, critics wrote mediocre reviews, citing *Mike & Molly*'s reliance on fat jokes. For instance, at the diner frequented by Mike and his police partner, Carl, the waiter refers to Mike as a "large man" and "big and bountiful." Carl also quips that he would shoot Mike if it weren't for not having enough chalk to outline Mike's large corpse. Later Carl hugs Mike while commenting, "It's like hugging a futon." Similarly, the pilot depicts Molly exercising on an elliptical machine while her mother eats a giant piece of chocolate cake and relaxes on the couch. After discussing Molly's lack of love life, her mother implores Molly's sister, "Why don't you take her to one of those lesbo clubs? They seem to like the beefy gals!" These types of jokes fill the first few episodes, with both Mike and Molly joking at their own expense as well as their family members and friends commenting about their body sizes.

A critic for ABC News, Coeli Carr, worried about the fat jokes being offensive, as did reviewers Kevin Fallon from the *Atlantic* and Joel Keller of the *Huffington Post*.[39] The predominance of fat jokes throughout the first few episodes of *Mike & Molly* even inspired *Movieline* to start a "Fat Joke Tracker" for the series, noting that in a single episode both Mike's body and Molly's are compared to a UPS truck, the cartoon character Shrek, an elephant, and an IMAX screen.[40] Across each review of *Mike & Molly* there is, given the prevalence of fat stigmatization and discrimination throughout society at large, an almost surprising amount of sensitivity concerning stereotypes of fat embodiment.

However, as *Mike & Molly* progresses, fat jokes become less frequent and both Mike and Molly develop as characters who happen to be fat as opposed to fat-focused characters, or in other words, fatness is less important to their overall identities, character developments, and interpersonal relationships. In fact, *Mike & Molly* actually goes a long way toward resisting and challenging fat stereotypes, namely that fat individuals are lazy, stupid, or ugly,[41] and its body politics exist in clear contrast to the depictions of fat self-loathing common across *The*

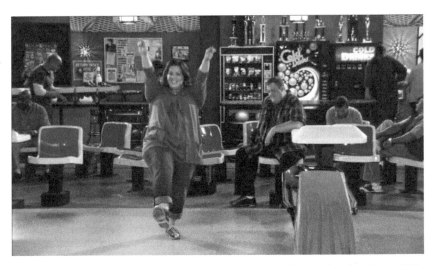

Figure 13   Mike and Molly bowling on the "First Kiss" episode of *Mike & Molly* (2010)

Biggest Loser and other weight-loss programs. Furthermore, and contrary to health and medicalized discourses, both Mike and Molly are not waiting to "start" their lives, fall in love, or achieve their goals until after they lose weight. As Mike, Molly, and all of the secondary characters develop throughout the series, Mike and Molly are portrayed as the most identifiable, "normal," success- ful, and rational, while their families and friends are one-dimensional caricatures rather than relatable, well-rounded characters. Molly is sweet, caring, intelligent, and funny, and Mike is kind, hardworking, and humorous. Comparatively, Mol- ly's thin and conventionally beautiful sister, Victoria, is unintelligent, unlucky in love with the already-married men she dates, a frequent drug user, and a beauti- cian at a funeral home (this career choice is played for comedy). Molly's mother, Joyce, is obsessed with staying youthful, has a quick temper, and drinks alcohol to excess. Mike's mother, Margaret (or "Peggy"), is cruel and demanding, and her only companion appears to be her dog.

Even though most episodes beyond the first few deal minimally with weight or fatness, the few that do are less stereotypical and more thoughtful explora- tions of experiencing fatness. At one Overeaters Anonymous meeting during an episode in the second season, "Mike Cheats," Mike is worried because he has been cheating on his diet, which he believes is preventing weight loss. There are, of course, a few fat jokes, including Carl telling Mike to jump in the clothes dryer with his shirt so he shrinks, and Mike saying to Carl about Molly, "She lost three pounds last week and all I lost is a Nutter Butter in the shower." Yet the narrative arc of the episode is one familiar to many who do attempt to lose weight. Mike eventually shares his food difficulties with Molly, explaining to her their relationship made him so happy that he let his guard down around food, which led to Mike eating more, feeling guilty about eating more, and then eating out of guilt, a cycle causing him to gain instead of lose weight. Molly shows compassion and understanding as Mike shares this all-too-common experience, and they decide to go to an Overeaters Anonymous meeting together, leaving Molly's home hand in hand. The episode concludes with a more serious tone than the show often does; Mike stands in front of the support group and says, "My name is Mike and I'm an overeater" as the scene fades to black. While this episode may reinforce the idea that fat individuals are fat because they overeat or all fat individuals have difficulty restraining themselves around food, the experience likely rings true for some individuals who do believe they overeat or have addictive relationships with food. In this sense, the show cannot be faulted for not being representative of the "fat experience" as there is no singular "fat experience," but instead various experiences and individualized feelings and relationships with one's own body.

Another episode in the second season, "The Dress," tells the story of Molly trying to lose six pounds in order to fit into her wedding dress prior to her wedding to Mike. To shed some weight, Molly shifts her diet into "overdrive" and basically begins starving herself (despite her sister recommending the "weight-loss miracle known as horse laxatives"). Fitting with the TV trope that dieting leads to impulsive or irrational behavior, Molly begins acting strangely and becomes short-tempered with everyone around her. At a spin class in the next scene, Molly runs into an old friend, who advises, "if you starve yourself you just gain more weight." Upset by the advice, Molly heads to her car while maniacally and angrily mumbling to herself, "Smug. Tiny Ass. One Chin." She begins frantically searching for candy in Mike's car, and upon finding some hidden in the glove compartment she immediately puts it in her mouth only to spit it out a moment later, saying out loud to herself, "Thought you had me this time, you fun size son of a bitch." Mike then joins Molly in the parking lot and they discuss Molly's erratic behavior and mood swings while dieting, or rather, not eating. Mike reassures Molly she already looks beautiful, saying, "You don't have to squeeze into some wedding dress to look perfect to me." In this episode, then, Molly's fat body is not the "problem"; the problem is the pressure Molly feels to be smaller on her wedding day, and the pressure to make her body fit into a garment rather than make a garment fit her body.

The critical response shifted later in the show's tenure, likely a result of the show's writers reducing the number of fat jokes. For example, one critic says, "*Mike & Molly* is a mushy and human exploration of the struggle to find pleasure away from the bakery aisle, and the fight fat people wage against objectification."[42] Similarly, David Hickley, a critic for *New York Daily News*, praised the show in his 2010 article: "The most promising thing about "Mike & Molly," in the bigger picture, is that they both like themselves. They'd prefer to be thinner, but their size isn't making them sit out of the dance. They're funny and engaging, and in the end, the size of their waists matters far less than the size of their hearts."[43] Melissa McCarthy echoes a similar sentiment in regard to the show not focusing on weight, further explaining why she loved the concept after reading the script: "I thought it had such lovely relationships, not just Billy at the beginning, but also my character's family, as crazy as it is. I love that this show doesn't have any snarky quality to it, but is still funny and lovely. If we lose weight, if we gain weight—that's just not the axis the show revolves around."[44] In regard to any lingering fat jokes on the show, Chuck Lorre offers his usual defense against potentially offensive comedy, which is basically one of comedic pluralism that does not take into account differences in power or status, saying, "There are fat jokes, but there are also booze jokes and tramp jokes. It's a show that spoofs all sorts of stereotypes. Nobody's sacred." However, Lorre emphasizes that the tone *Mike & Molly* uses in regard to all of its jokes, but particularly fat jokes, is important, adding, "The truth without love is abuse," and that *Mike & Molly* "is coming from a caring place, not a hurtful place."[45]

While a majority of body-positive programs are scripted, unlike those discussed in previous chapters, there are several reality programs engaging with fat positivity and acceptance. For instance, Fox's short-lived *More to Love* is a dating show for fat women that markets itself as a "progressive portrayal of real women," but reifies fatness as a problem or source of anguish for most of the show's participants.[46] Two other examples include *Ruby* on the Style Network and *Chelsea Settles* (2011) on MTV. Both programs represent fat women who desire and actively work toward losing weight, but like *Drop Dead Diva*, *Huge*, and *Mike & Molly*, each show ultimately focuses more on other aspects of these women's lives, including their romantic relationships, friendships, and careers. While these two programs do reinforce weight loss as necessary and desirable, they simultaneously counter fat stereotypes in the sense that both featured women who are physically active, generally happy and confident, and working toward achieving a variety of goals as opposed to putting life "on hold" until after they lose weight.

Moreover, *Big Sexy* and *Curvy Girls* are perhaps the most fat-positive reality television programs. Both TV series feature "plus-size" women working in the fashion industry as models, designers, or makeup artists. Both *Big Sexy* and *Curvy Girls* also resist many fat stereotypes and binary assumptions about thin versus fat women, portraying a wide array of fat body shapes and sizes. All of the women on both series are beautifully and fashionably styled and professionally successful, lead active social lives, and exude confidence not just despite the fact that they are fat, but also because they love their fat bodies. The women of *Big Sexy*, in particular, engage in several activities defying the idea that life begins post–weight loss, including hosting a plus-size bikini fashion show, pole dancing for aerobic exercise, and vajazzling. In fact, one *Big Sexy* character, Leslie Medlik, a fashion stylist, even addresses this during the show's introduction, saying, "If you think I'm going to sit in my room and hide cause I'm not a size 2, you're crazy!"

The series' characters do not talk about weight in relation to health, and with the exception of one episode of season 2 of *Curvy Girls* in which Rosie thinks losing weight will help her book more modeling gigs, they almost never talk about weight loss. Instead they work out and eat in order to maintain their current weights—which would classify them as obese according to the body mass index. Executive producers of both *Curvy Girls* and *Big Sexy* say they actively avoid conversations about health and weight loss in order to explicitly offer alternative programming. Bruce David Klein, the executive producer of *Big Sexy*, explains, "It was very purposeful. This was always about women who were comfortable with their size. Of course we explored the consequences of their size in a range of scenes—but weight loss was never part of the conversation—too many other shows deal in that space and we wanted to show another side."[47] The consequences Klein is referring to include not getting modeling jobs as an "in-betweener" and scenes where the women are in public and strangers are hostile, gawk at them, or comment on their bodies. In this sense, *Big Sexy* and *Curvy Girls* embrace fat acceptance and explore various fat experiences, showing that many of the difficulties of fat embodiment stem not from just being fat, but rather from the interpersonal relationships and interactions influenced by particular cultural and social contexts as well as public health and medical discourses.

Tiffany Banks, one of the models featured on *Big Sexy*, speaks openly about the body-positive and fat-positive goals of the program within the context of the obesity epidemic: "We were trying to make plus-size women visible in a positive light, which I think we accomplished. We made sure we showed that we all have active lifestyles and that we are focused on being healthy, both physically and mentally. We worked out, did fun physical activities like pole dancing class and boxing, and were active. Had we had more time on air we would have gotten more in depth but I made sure when signing on that we emphasized that being plus size doesn't necessarily mean that you are unhealthy."[48] Both *Big Sexy* and *Curvy Girls* can perhaps be considered the antithesis of *The Biggest Loser* or *My 600-lb Life* in terms of both the way fatness itself is framed (something to celebrate versus something to abhor) and the way fat individuals are generally represented (happy with themselves versus a thin *person* "trapped" in a fat *body*). These overt differences in the way television represents fatness and fat experiences, namely that *Big Sexy* and *Curvy Girls* portray an alternative to fat hate and fat stigmatization still rare on television and other mainstream information and entertainment outlets, likely explains the short-lived nature of both programs. *Big Sexy* lasted only three episodes despite creating tremendous buzz for TLC on fat-acceptance

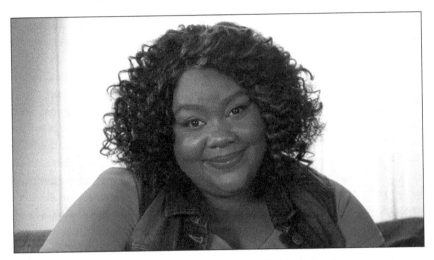

Figure 14   Nicole on *Loosely Exactly Nicole* (2016)

forums. *Curvy Girls* lasted a bit longer, making it two short seasons, but on NuvoTV, a small cable channel marketed toward bicultural Latinos living in the United States. But less important than audience scope or program longevity is the fact that TV shows with overt body-/fat-positive messages demonstrate the increasing social acceptability of different fat narratives.

Another short-lived show, MTV's *Loosely Exactly Nicole* (2017), takes the opposite approach to representing fat acceptance. Instead of directly addressing fatness like the participants of *Big Sexy* and *Curvy Girls*, *Loosely Exactly Nicole* opts for its main character to be a fully formed fat character rather than one focusing on her fatness. Nicole Byer explains the uniqueness of this approach: "A fat Black lady who just fucks people left and right on her show, and we never talk about how she's fat and Black? That's crazy!"[49] Of course it makes sense for the participants of *Big Sexy* and *Curvy Girls* to place so much emphasis on bodies, as that is what the fashion and beauty industry is focused on and their bodies are their livelihoods. Ultimately, just like *Girls* and *The Mindy Project*, both kinds of representations are important, and their copresence is even more important. We need to directly address fatness while also representing fatness as just another type of embodiment rather than an all-consuming aspect of one's identity. Byer argues, "I look at women like Queen Latifah, Monique and Gabourey Sidibe as having paved the way for someone like me to exist. So, *Living Single*, *The Parkers*— without these shows, I wouldn't have my show." And she's right. The more fat representation we have on television, the more varied those fat representation will be, and the less of a representational burden each fat character will shoulder.

Conclusion

None of the texts discussed in this chapter are politically or socially perfect, and what "perfection" could even mean is both questionable and unattainable. I am less interested in what each of these texts does that is "good" or "bad," opting instead for a reparative reading of superficially problematic texts. Instead of random sitcom episodes about characters dieting or flashbacks to when a character used to be fat, there are now sustained representations and discussions of a wider variety of bodies across television. Some critiques over the limited representational range of fat embodiment are fair, but as more fat individuals are featured on the small screen, such as on programs like NBC's *This Is Us* (2016–), ABC's *American Housewife* (2016–), AMC's *Dietland* (2018–), and Netflix's *Glow* (2017–) the representational burden each reality TV participant or TV character carries will undoubtedly lessen.

The fat-acceptance discourses taken up in many of these television texts play with and resist how fat people are both individualized and massified according to public health and medical institutions and experts. A primary aspect of both fat acceptance and body size diversity is to resist the ways in which fatness is used to categorize people into populations in need of monitoring and intervention or treatment. By focusing less on the medical and health aspects of the body, body- and fat-positive TV programs assert fat individuals as *actual people*. The reality participants and characters across theses series are considered people who have partners, jobs, families, and issues of concern outside the size of their bodies. And for the most part, their health statuses do not matter. These representations and narratives, then, challenge fat stereotypes and fat phobia throughout the United States by contributing to the visual diversity of bodies and multiplicity of fat experiences on the small screen. Additionally, these programs also resist the individualizing aspects of health and medical discourses of fatness. Instead of reinforcing the notion that fat individuals lack the necessary self-discipline or self-control to lose weight or that fat individuals are lazy and unhappy with their bodies, these TV programs represent different kinds of fat attitudes, ones more likely to encourage positivity, self-acceptance, and maybe even self-love.

A Note on Policy

Currently, discussions of body and fat positivity reflecting discourses of fat acceptance are not present in communication or health policy debates. These ideas may yet be too outside of mainstream health and medical thought to fit within the current discursive rules and frameworks used by regulatory bodies. Thomas Streeter argues that discursive rules within regulatory interpretative communities determine what sense is made of particular ideas or whether they are brought up at all. Streeter contends that regulatory bodies, like all interpretive communities, develop their own shared understandings and assumptions, which can limit the scope of policy debates while still allowing for slow change over time in response to particular technological, industrial, and social contexts.[50] So whereas chapters 2 and 3 demonstrate the interplay between communication policies and industry practices and representations and chapter 4 looks at health policies and organizations in relation to medicalized bodies, the fat-acceptance discourses and emerging industry lore discussed in this chapter are, perhaps, only beginning to open a discursive space for health regulators, specifically, to consider Health at Every Size (HAES) or notions of fat acceptance in obesity epidemic debates. But as body and fat positivity become more prevalent on television and public health interventions and medical treatments continue failing, while simultaneously promoting fat stigmatization, it's likely HAES and aspects of fat acceptance will be welcomed in policy spheres in the future. For instance, the National Institutes of Health held a panel on obesity in 1992, and while HAES was not specifically mentioned (as it was not yet developed), the panel's recommendation aligns with the approach: "A focus on approaches that produce health benefits independently of weight loss may be the best way to improve the physical and psychological health of Americans seeking to lose weight."

Conclusion

THE DECLINE OF
THE BIGGEST LOSER

As alternative stories of fat embodiment become more common on television, producers of shows like *The Biggest Loser* are finding it harder to manage the continual and even intensifying criticism. In the fall of 2009, *The Biggest Loser* was already drawing heavy disapproval after a former contestant admitted to dropping weight by fasting and dehydrating himself to the point of urinating blood, while another admitted to fasting and working out in multiple layers of clothing when the cameras were turned off.[1] Kai Hibbard, a finalist on the third season of *The Biggest Loser*, reveals that contestants were forced against doctors' orders to work out through injuries and were advised to dehydrate themselves before weigh-ins in order to achieve bigger weight-loss numbers. Hibbard also says she developed disordered eating practices while participating on the show, which continued for years afterward.[2] Another participant, Suzanne Mendonca, says she was forced to exercise despite stress fractures in her feet, further claiming contestants would spend hours a day in saunas, wrap themselves in garbage bags to increase sweat production when exercising, and would even stop eating and drinking entirely before weigh-ins.[3] And yet another participant, Lezlye Donahue (season 4), says she was actually encouraged to gain some weight before appearing on the show because she was deemed not quite big enough for weight-loss TV. Donahue feels manipulated by the show, saying that going on *The Biggest Loser* was a worse experience for her than surviving Hurricane Katrina.[4] Finally, another participant, Joelle Gwyn (season 7), claims the show provided her with ephedra, a dangerous and largely banned substance used for "energy" and appetite suppression, leading the Los Angeles Sheriff's Department to open an inquiry into the allegations.[5]

Bob Harper and Dr. Huizinga unequivocally denied these claims, with Huizinga saying, "These allegations are absolutely false and are in direct conflict with my lifelong devotion to health and fitness."[6] Some past participants of the show also took to social media to deny the claims of their fellow contestants, but it's ultimately difficult to know the extent or severity of these kinds of experiences because contestants are not allowed to talk to reporters without permission from the show. And when they do talk to reporters their discussions are closely monitored. In fact, one of the talent producers for *The Biggest Loser* wrote in an

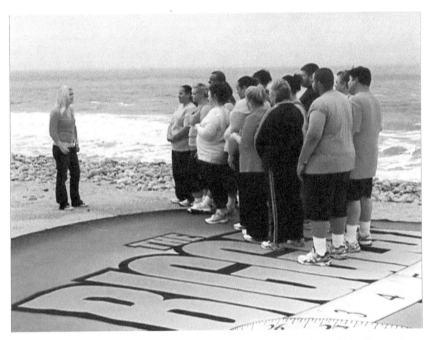

Figure 15   The "second chance" workout on season 8, episode 1 of *The Biggest Loser* (2009)

email to a former participant that talking to reporters could result in a fine ranging from a hundred thousand to a million dollars.[7] Despite this highly controlled messaging, participant experiences are mostly corroborated by depictions on the show itself, with the 2013 season arc incorporating the controversy of Jillian Michaels giving her team caffeine pills to help them lose more weight.[8]

Even if we cannot yet know the extent of the practices taking place behind the scenes, what is exhibited on-screen already generates a significant amount of criticism. *The Biggest Loser* is referred to as an "emotionally and physically abusive, misinformative, horror show" by physician Yoni Freedhoff, who also critiques the show's practices as detrimental to participants maintaining long-term weight loss because high-intensity workouts lasting six to eight hours each day combined with overly restrictive diets "decimates" the metabolism.[9] Freedhoff adds that this makes participants more likely to gain weight after the show, which substantiates claims made by three alumni of *The Biggest Loser* who assert 85 to 90 percent of participants on the show regain their lost weight. Similarly, Michael Mantell, a fitness consultant, argues that *The Biggest Loser* is "unsafe, ineffective, and downright demotivating for many. . . . The reality is that the show is not reality and does not represent a weight-loss program as it should be or can be pursued by a vast majority of people."[10] The practices on the show lead to one writer making the case for the necessity of a disclaimer before the opening credits of each episode: "Warning: This show documents dangerous ideas and behavior that can, if taken seriously and copied, result in physical and emotional trauma, and risks serious permanent injury including death. It will not help you to learn how to solve your weight problem and may make it worse."[11]

One study documenting the health and weight statuses of former participants of *The Biggest Loser* paints a bleak picture of the body's ability to sustain significant weight loss.[12] Kevin Hall, a researcher at the National Institutes of Health and lead author of the study, found that participants had significantly lower metabolisms post–weight loss and that their metabolisms not only failed to recover but actually continued to slow over time. In fact, Danny Cahill's metabolism slowed to the point that he can eat only eight hundred calories per day just to *maintain* his weight of 295 pounds. Based on these findings, the study's authors argue, "Even the most motivated are working against their own biology." Another takeaway from these findings? "The difficulty in keeping weight off reflects biology, not a pathological lack of willpower affecting two-thirds of the U.S.A."[13]

In response to this study, J. D. Roth, executive producer of *The Biggest Loser*, argues that the actual weight-gain statistic for the show's participants is around 50 percent, adding, "Getting one hundred percent to keep the weight off has never been the goal. . . . The goal is can we inspire people in America to make a change in their life. In that, we're batting a thousand."[14] And to demonstrate that the 50 percent of individuals who do regain do so because of their individual choices—or their "pathological lack of willpower"—rather than their slowed metabolism, he created a new weight-loss series airing on the small cable channel Z Living: *The Big Fat Truth* (2017). The show, which is essentially a public relations attempt to restore the integrity of *The Biggest Loser* while promoting Roth's new weight-loss book of the same name, features former participants of *The Biggest Loser* who have all regained a significant amount of weight since being on the show (further demonstrating the disciplinary discrepancies and failures of these weight loss series). Ramon (season 12) gained 153 pounds, Ryan (season 1) 124 pounds, Tiffany (season 4) 70 pounds, and Mallory (season 5) 80 pounds. Two other participants on Roth's *The Big Fat Truth* actually now weigh more than they did before appearing on *The Biggest Loser*, with Curtis (season 5) gaining 175 pounds and Jessica (season 12) 149 pounds. The participants discuss the individual reasons why they gained weight, but each story is along the same lines as Mallory explaining that she just did not stick to her diet and kept "self-destructing." Summarizing their stories, Roth concludes, "Their old habits crept back in."

Roth again rhetorically asks participants of *The Big Fat Truth*, "Is it your metabolism? Or is it your choices?" Roth then uses the show to "prove" to us it's the latter—weight is choice—while also providing us with another example of the way he's "proved" science "wrong." He first "proved" science "wrong" in regard to the amount of weight individuals can or should lose every week, with most medical doctors arguing that one to two pounds a *week* is sustainable.

However, *The Biggest Loser* pushed contestants to lose one to two pounds per *day*. Roth details how he was able to "defeat the scientific part" in the past: "So that one-two pounds a week turns into double-digit weight loss every week. We had people losing ten pounds a week, several weeks in a row—and that's not because I'm better or smarter than doctors—because I don't even have a college degree. It's just because I play the game of the mind. If you fix your mind, your body follows."[15] Roth ultimately says that he just does not *believe* the widely shared metabolic study to be true, that he does not *believe* weight is a matter of biology or physiology.[16] Instead, *The Big Fat Truth* pushes a low-calorie, plant-based diet and focuses on behavioral and emotional issues, while Roth repeatedly says (as if the more often he repeats it the more likely it will be true), "It's not your metabolism. It's your head." Of course *The Big Fat Truth* just like *The Biggest Loser* reinforces "a dangerous approach to weight loss that favors quick results over science."[17]

The Biggest Loser is not alone in receiving criticism for its weight-loss practices. A participant on the first season of *Extreme Weight Loss*, James Garrison, posted on his personal blog (since removed) that he experienced numerous medical problems both while on the show and afterward due to losing such a large amount of body weight in such a small amount of time. Garrison says he asked *Extreme Weight Loss* for help paying his medical bills, but after receiving cease and desist letters from ABC's legal department instead of the help he wanted, he decided to "blow the whistle" on the show's practices. Garrison wrote on his blog that he was instructed to dehydrate himself prior to weigh-ins and to take diet pills (similar to accusations against *The Biggest Loser*), adding that he saw the show's host and trainer only a few times that entire year (countering the show's assertion that Powell moves in with each participant for the first three months of their transformations).

These kinds of high-profile controversies—and subsequent uninspiring and see-through public relations attempts by J. D. Roth—mark a potential turning point in the way we talk about and televise fat narratives and representations. Narratives of weight loss are not likely on the way out, or at least not yet, but rather may be becoming more complex and more compassionate as more of these shows are exposed as ineffective and counterproductive to their stated health goals

As this project hopefully demonstrates, fat television exists in multiple forms and offers multiple messages about the body, both within the series themselves and across them. Some series focus on weight loss, others on the medicalization of fat bodies in relation to disease, and others still on encouraging body positivity or fat acceptance. Each set of texts is articulated to particular discourses of the body, and those discourses of the body are circulated, legitimized, and negotiated by news organizations and social media accounts as well as various regulatory bodies and organizations, from the FCC to WHO. These discourses of the body, which are always already terrains of struggle, are taken up by and further destabilized and debated across television texts. Thus, while television reinforces dominant discourses serving dominant social and political interests in the context of neoliberalism and the obesity epidemic, it still negotiates and sometimes undermines those very discourses and operates as a site of multidiscursivity.

Furthermore, television can be thought of in a variety of ways, all of which are important to this project, including as a surveillance appendage that governs, disciplines, and controls at a distance, as way to generate capital for corporations, as working in service of the public interest, as a vehicle for medicalization, as a hegemonic process with instances of resistance, and as an asynchronous cultural forum that weaves together various ways of thinking about fatness, health, and the body. All of these competing and copresent understandings of television must be taken into consideration as we theorize power, discipline, and control, yet reality television scholarship, specifically, fails to account for many of these important aspects of TV. Yes, television may work to govern at a distance and discipline those on-screen as well as those at home, but it also exposes its own inability to effectively govern, discipline, and transform citizens at a distance because it is, fundamentally, a polysemic and multidiscursive medium that is influenced by the various politics and interests of program creators, by both dominant and emerging industry lore, by medical, health, and body activist understandings of the fat body, and by regulators as well as governmental and nongovernmental organizations. Even as television changes through channel proliferation, content migration, and distribution flexibility and as society itself shifts, splinters, or unites, the texts we encounter are still complex, contingent, and articulated to various terrains of struggle and competing interests.

For example, discourses across these different fat television texts are also now colliding and interacting in interesting ways. Jillian Michaels, who is best known as a weight-loss trainer on *The Biggest Loser*, recently defended *Mike & Molly*'s Melissa McCarthy on an episode of *Entertainment Tonight* after a film critic, Rex Reed, called her "tractor-sized" and a "female hippo." Michaels labeled Reed's comments "cruel" and "evil," saying that they not only are hurtful to "plus-size" women, but also lead to discrimination against large people. It's somewhat ironic for Michaels to talk about cruelty as she is known for constantly berating participants on *The Biggest Loser* and supporting a commercial entity that arguably accomplishes little more than reinforcing fat stigmatization. But Michaels's final words on the *ET* segment, specifically that she is more concerned about health than weight, are reminiscent of fat-acceptance discourses more so than current health and medicalized discourses within the context of the obesity epidemic. Thus, one of the United States' biggest, most well-known advocates for weight loss is now deemphasizing the numbers on a scale, which will arguably mitigate her notoriety for saying similarly hurtful comments to dozens of contestants over the years on *The Biggest Loser*.

This overlap is also present across this book's chapters despite their discursive categorizations. Although narratives and representations on *Mike & Molly* reinforce the desirability of weight loss in accordance with health discourses, both characters refuse to let their fatness prevent them from living, which is far more body- and fat-positive than reality weight-loss shows. The characters of Mike and Molly both have good careers and loving relationships and set out to achieve their goals, evidenced by Molly deciding to apply to the prestigious Iowa Writer's Workshop in the show's fourth season. The television series *Ruby* (2008– 2011), which aired for multiple seasons on the Style network, also represents this discursive convergence. After experiencing physical impairment and social disability at her highest weight of 715 pounds, Ruby seeks medical treatment, specifically psychiatry, and loses 400 pounds through controlled eating via a surveilling nursing staff. Following the weight loss, Ruby then diets and increases her physical activity under the supervision of nutritionists and trainers. These common practices that reinforce notions of self-discipline or self-control also integrate medical treatment, combing health and medicalized understandings of the fat body. And throughout her health and medicalized weight-loss journey, Ruby travels, has romantic partners, bonds with her friends and family, and generally has a positive outlook on life and a self-accepting attitude about her body. Like shows articulated to body positivity or fat acceptance, life does not stop because of fatness. *Ruby* thus weaves health, medicalized, and fat-acceptance discourses of the body into one series, demonstrating them all to be relevant and important to her lived experience as a fat woman. *Ruby* reminds us that none of these TV series exist in isolation from each other, and while particular discourses more strongly influence particular sets of texts, creating an asynchronous cultural forum rather than just a surveillance appendage that disciplines and controls, they are also articulated to each other through their fat visibilities. These texts, then, are always understood in relation to other TV texts and the social, industrial, regulatory, and health or medical contexts from which they emerge and which they influence.

In consideration of these overlaps and articulations, one important direction for future research is to examine whether those who watch *The Biggest Loser* also watch *Curvy Girls*. Are viewers of these programs fat TV omnivores, like myself, or do they primarily watch one type of fat television or certain channels that exhibit a particular kind of fat programming? In other words, are viewers being exposed to all of these discourses of the fat body, beyond their inherent overlaps, or are they choosing the programs that most closely align with their own body politics? Another direction for future research is to more fully explore the production context through interviews. What are the goals or motivations behind particular narrative and representational choices? Did producers of *Curvy Girls*, *Big Sexy*, and *Huge* receive pushback from their channel or network executives? What types of representational compromises were made, if any? Interviews with program creators as well as regulators and advertisers could more fully elucidate how various fat discourses traverse, clash, and coexist throughout the circuit of culture.

Theories of intersectionality also need to be considered more thoroughly in order to understand how fatness is both experienced and read differently based on overlapping aspects of our identities, locations, and systems of oppression. Fat Black bodies are often socially positioned and read in differing ways than fat white bodies; fat men and women also experience fatness differently. Even though discourses of globesity demonstrate just how widespread fat stigma may be around the world, fatness is still constitutive of various cultural influences and national or regional contexts. Gay men arguably experience fatness differently than straight men, which makes Cam and Mitchell's bodily diverse relationship on *Modern Family* a potential site to explore the intersectionality of fatness, sexuality, and the "tyranny of buffness" within gay communities.[18]

We may also inscribe different attributes and characteristics to fat middle- or upper-class bodies in comparison to working-class bodies. Governor Chris Christie, Oprah, and other political leaders, celebrities, and members of the wealthy elite who publicly "struggle" with fatness both experience fatness differently and have their fatness interpreted differently due to their economic and social statuses. Do wealthy fat individuals complicate assumptions connecting fatness and class to the eating of processed, low-quality foods or the watching of television as a cause of the obesity epidemic? Do wealthy fat individuals complicate the "common sense" solutions of diet, exercise, and surgical interventions being successful for weight loss considering the fact that these individuals can pay for high-quality food, physical trainers, and surgery, yet they continue to embody fatness? Is it possible that fat individuals who are wealthy somehow simultaneously receive more and less judgment because of their class status? In other words, despite limitless resources, they may be especially viewed as, allegedly, lacking the self-discipline or self-control "necessary" to lose weight, yet their fatness may be blamed less on typical fat stereotypes like laziness or stupidity given their other financial and social success, or status as otherwise good neoliberal subjects. Just for these reasons alone, we need to consider the way multiple identity categories and contexts work together to constitute understandings and experiences, including oppressions and celebrations, of fat bodies.

In the future, we also need to more closely examine the way televised constructions of health in relation to fatness employ, according to Jonathan Metzl, a "language of betterment, skillfully glossing over issues of moralism, sexism, classism, racism and other 'isms' that may be present in news reporting, public health campaigns," and, for our purposes, television programs.[19] Although this project only begins to scratch the surface of the relationship between television and fatness, or between communication and health policies, media industries, and fat representations and narratives, it illustrates both the complex and important nature of those relationships in how we understand television itself and fatness within the context of the obesity epidemic.

Ultimately, each of these areas of fat television will undoubtedly continue to develop in different ways and in tandem with the allegedly expanding waistlines of citizens around the world. Even though most fat TV programs work to reinforce the necessity and desirability of weight loss rather than promoting body positivity or fat acceptance, shows engaging with alternative as well as intrinsically and overtly resistant representations and narratives of the body are now more frequent and wider in reach than they were when I started this project several years ago. Television shows that embrace body size diversity through fat visibility or address the various ways fatness is experienced and understood will endure as the context of the obesity epidemic heightens concern over our bodies and fatness. While the obesity epidemic is simultaneously constructed and deconstructed by television, fat representations and narratives require us to consider television as an asynchronous cultural forum, as a contradictory medium of discipline, medicalization, information, entertainment, and maybe even fat resistance.

Acknowledgments

I am grateful to so many people who contributed both to this book and to my development as a media scholar. I started this project as a graduate student in the Department of Communication Studies at the University of Iowa, where I was supported and challenged by smart and inspiring professors and colleagues in classes, in department seminars, and while lingering in the halls of Becker. They include Timothy Havens, Rita Zajacz, Joy Hayes, M. Gigi Durham, Kembrew McLeod, Mark Andrejevic, John Durham Peters, Isaac West, Jeff Bennett, Leslie Baxter, Adam Rugg, Michaela Frischherz, Lindsey Thomas, Rebecca Robinson Chávez, Brook Irving, Dan Faltesek, Lauren-Ashley Buchanan, Benjamin Burroughs, Ben Morton, Josh Pederson, and Laurena Bernabo.

I owe a lot of this book to my forever-advisor, Elana Levine, who continues to support me even though I stopped being her student a long time ago. My colleagues and friends at Merrimack College, especially Lisa Perks, Jacob Turner, Andrew Tollison, and Sam Bruno, are never-ending in their encouragement and wonderfully snarky commentary. I am indebted to my friend and fellow feminist scholar, Raechel Tiffe, for the frequent work dates and her invaluable feedback on a draft of this book. I would also like to thank Laura Portwood-Stacer and Manuscript Works for guidance in transforming this project from a dissertation to a book. Both the University of Iowa and Merrimack College provided me with financial support through fellowships and grants at different stages of this project. Additionally, I am grateful for all of the feedback from my editor at Rutgers University Press, Lisa Banning, the anonymous reviewers at different stages of this project, and Esther Rothblum and Kathleen LeBesco.

Finally, I would like to thank my parents, Tom and Karla Zimdars, for far too many things to list here. And to John Bittrich, my partner, proofreader, and fellow TV-marathoner: I'll never be able to thank you enough for your patience, kindness, and support.

Notes

CHAPTER 1 — TELEVISING FATNESS

1. Harriet Brown, *Body of Truth: How Science, History, and Culture Drive Our Obsession with Weight—And What We Can Do about It* (Boston: De Capo Press, 2015).

2. Abigail Saguy, *What's Wrong with Fat?* (Oxford: Oxford University Press, 2013), 15.

3. Sharlene Nagy Hesse-Biber argues that this common "pursuit of thinness" is a primary or fundamental concern for many women because they are encouraged from a young age to connect the idea of self-worth to the ability to attract a partner, and body weight is seen as an important component of physical attraction. See Sharlene Nagy Hesse-Biber, *The Cult of Thinness* (Oxford: Oxford University Press, 2006).

4. Roberta Sassatelli, *Fitness Culture: Gyms and the Commercialisation of Discipline and Fun* (New York: Palgrave Macmillan, 2010).

5. Susie Orbach, *Fat Is a Feminist Issue* (New York: Berkley Books, 1978).

6. "Health" is a vague and all-encompassing term that is incredibly hard to define. We generally think of health as something positive or a desired state of being, but Jonathan M. Metzl notes that it is a contested term, and one that is also a "prescribed state and an ideological position." See Jonathan M. Metzl, "Introduction: Why 'Against Health'?," in *Against Health: How Health Became the New Morality*, ed. Jonathan M. Metzl and Anna Kirkland (New York: New York University Press, 2010), 1–2.

7. Hélène Joffe and Staerklé, "The Centrality of the Self-Control Ethos in Western Aspersions Regarding Outgroups: A Social Representational Approach to Stereotype Content," *Culture & Psychology* 13, no. 4 (2007): 405.

8. Toby Miller, *Cultural Citizenship: Cosmopolitanism, Consumerism, and Television in the Neoliberal Age* (Philadelphia: Temple University Press, 2007); Laurie Ouellette, "Take Responsibility for Yourself: *Judge Judy* and the Neoliberal Citizen," in *Feminist Television Criticism: A Reader*, ed. Charlotte Brunsdon and Lynn Spigel (Berkshire: Open University Press, 2008), 151.

9. Elana Levine, *Wallowing in Sex: The New Sexual Culture of 1970s American Television* (Durham, N.C.: Duke University Press, 2007), 6.

10. Ron Becker, *Gay TV and Straight America* (New Brunswick, N.J.: Rutgers University Press, 2006), 11.

11. Herman Gray, *Watching Race: Television and the Struggle for "Blackness"* (Minneapolis: University of Minnesota Press, 1995), 7.

12. Amy Gullage, "Fat Monica, Fat Suits, and *Friends*," *Feminist Media Studies* 14, no. 2 (2014): 178–189.

13. Lily Kalin, "Want to Know How You Can Tell Our Culture Is Fat Phobic? Watch TV," *Huffington Post*, October 10, 2014, www.huffingtonpost.com/2014/10/10/formerly-fat-tv-trope _n_5962704.html; Katharina R. Mendoza, "Seeing through the Layers: Fat Suits and Thin Bodies in *The Nutty Professor* and *Shallow Hal*," in *The Fat Studies Reader*, ed. Esther Rothblum and Sondra Solovay (New York: New York University Press, 2009), 280–288.

14. Jerry Mosher, "Setting Free the Bears: Refiguring Fat Men on Television," in *Bodies Out of Bounds: Fatness and Transgression*, ed. Jana Evans Braziel and Kathleen LeBesco (Berkeley: University of California Press, 2001), 166–196.

15. To my knowledge, neither intersex fat characters nor fat transgender characters appear on television. I say this to acknowledge that sex and gender are not binaries in the same way that fat and thin should not be considered discrete binaries. The limitation is thus a reflection of the realities of current television representations rather than an oversight of the intersections of fatness, gender, and sex.

16. Mosher, "Setting Free the Bears."

17. Timothy Havens, "Guy-Coms and the Hegemony of Juvenile Masculinity." *Flow*, October 7, 2007, http://flowtv.org/2007/10/guy-coms-and-the-hegemony-of-juvenile-masculinity/; Matt Feeney, "Beauty and the Beast," *Slate*, January 5, 2005, www.slate.com/articles/arts/television/2005/01/beauty_and_the_beast.html.

18. J. Eric Oliver, *Fat Politics* (Oxford: Oxford University Press, 2006).

19. Sandra Lee Bartky, "Foucault, Femininity, and the Modernization of Patriarchal Power," in *The Politics of Women's Bodies: Sexuality, Appearance, and Behavior*, ed. Rose Weitz (Oxford: Oxford University Press 1998), 28, 80.

20. Bradley S. Greenberg, Matthew Eastin, Linda Hofschire, Ken Lachlan, and Kelly D. Brownell, "Portrayals of Overweight and Obese Individuals on Commercial Television," *American Journal of Public Health* 93 (2003): 1342–1348.

21. Bartky, "Foucault, Femininity, and the Modernization of Patriarchal Power," 63.

22. Cecilia Hartley, "Letting Ourselves Go: Making Room for the Fat Body in Feminist Scholarship," in Braziel and LeBesco, *Bodies Out of Bounds*, 67.

23. Bartky, "Foucault, Femininity, and the Modernization of Patriarchal Power," 35.

24. Gregory Fouts and Kimberly Burggraf, "Television Situation Comedies: Female Weight, Male Negative Comments, and Audience Reactions," *Sex Roles* 42, nos. 9–10 (1999): 925–932.

25. Dina Giovanelli and Stephen Osterag, "Controlling the Body: Media Representations, Body Size, and Self-Discipline," in Rothblum and Solovay, *Fat Studies Reader*, 289–299.

26. Beth Bernstein and Matilda St. John, "The Roseanne Benedict Arnolds: How Fat Women Are Betrayed by Their Celebrity Icons," in Rothblum and Solovay, *Fat Studies Reader*, 267.

27. The mammy figure is consistently desexualized so as not to "entice" the family patriarch, which itself reflects dubious assumptions about fatness, Blackness, and sexuality. Myrna A. Hant, "African American and Jewish Mothers/Wives on Television: Persistent Stereotypes," in *Media/Culture Studies: Critical Approaches*, ed. Rhonda Hammer and Douglas Kellner (New York: Peter Lang, 2009), 368.

28. Ibid.

29. Patricia Hill Collins, "Mammies, Matriarchs, and Other Controlling Images," in *Placing Women's Studies*, ed. Judith Raiskin, Roger Adkins, Shelley Kowalski, and Kathleen Sullivan (New York: McGraw-Hill, 1999), 124–125; bell hooks, *Ain't I a Woman* (Boston: South End Press, 1981), 8.

30. Amanda Lotz, "Using 'Network' Theory in a Post-network Era: Fictional 9/11 U.S. Television Discourse as a 'Cultural Forum,'" *Screen* 45, no. 4 (2004): 423–439.

31. Mark Andrejevic, *Reality TV: The Work of Being Watched* (New York: Rowman & Littlefield, 2004).

32. John Fiske, *Television Culture* (New York: Routledge, 1987), 154.

33. Dana Heller, "Intelligent Self-Design," *Television and New Media* 10, no. 1 (2009): 78.

34. Deborah Lupton, *Fat* (New York: Routledge, 2013), 3.

35. Louis J. Aronne, Donald S. Nelinson, and Joseph L. Lillo, "Obesity as a Disease State: A New Paradigm for Diagnosis and Treatment," *Clinical Cornerstone* 9, no. 4 (2009): 9–29.

CHAPTER 2 — COMPETING UNDERSTANDINGS OF FATNESS

1. Maura Kelly, "Should 'Fatties' Get a Room? (Even on TV?)," *Marie Claire*, October 25, 2010, www.marieclaire.com/sex-love/dating-blog/overweight-couples-on-television.

2. Hollie McKay, "Do Shows Focusing on Overweight Characters Further Obesity Problem?," *Fox News*, September 16, 2010, www.foxnews.com/entertainment/2010/09/16/shows -focusing-overweight-characters-obesity-problem/.

3. Coeli Carr, "TV's New Sitcom 'Mike & Molly': Are Fat Jokes Funny or Offensive?," *ABC News*, September 28, 2010, http://abcnews.go.com/Entertainment/mike-molly-fat-jokes -funny-offensive/story?id=11692329#.Ucx3Hvb8kt; Emily Exton, "Should 'Fatties' Get a Room? No. But It Is Time for TV to Move beyond the Fat Jokes," *Entertainment Weekly*, October 28, 2010, http://popwatch.ew.com/2010/10/28/marie-claire-fatties-mike-and-molly/; Alex Cohen, "Big, Fat Stereotypes Play Out on the Small Screen," *NPR*, August 8, 2011, www .npr.org/2011/08/08/138958386/big-fat-stereotypes-play-out-on-the-small-screen.

4. Rennie Dyball, *"My Big Fat Fabulous Life* Star: I'm Not Promoting Obesity," *People*, February 9, 2015, http://people.com/tv/my-big-fat-fabulous-life-star-whitney-thore-im-not-promoting -obesity/.

5. For a more thorough discussion of the various fat frames that exist, see Abigail Saguy, *What's Wrong with Fat?* (Oxford: Oxford University Press, 2013); Samantha Kwan and Jennifer Graves, *Framing Fat: Competing Constructions in Contemporary Culture* (New Brunswick, N.J.: Rutgers University Press, 2013).

6. The body mass index classifies individuals as "normal," "overweight," or "obese," among other categories, based on a height-to-weight ratio, but it is a poor indicator of one's overall health or body composition. For a comprehensive critique, see Paul Campos, *The Obesity Myth* (New York: Gotham Books, 2004).

7. World Health Organization, "Obesity and Overweight" (2018), www.who.int/mediacentre /factsheets/fs311/en/.

8. C. S. Li and R. Sinha, "Inhibitory Control and Emotional Stress Regulation: Neuroimaging Evidence for Frontal-Limbic Dysfunction in Psycho-Stimulant Addiction," *Neuroscience & Biobehavioral Reviews* 32 (2008): 581–597; J. Feil, D. Sheppard, P. B. Fitzgerald, M. Yücel, D. I. Lubman, D. I., and J. L. Bradshaw, "Addiction, Compulsive Drug Seeking, and the Role of Frontostriatal Mechanisms in Regulating Inhibitory Control," *Neuroscience & Biobehavioral Reviews* 35 (2010): 248–275; Maoyong Fan and Yanhong Jin, "Obesity and Self-Control: Food Consumption, Physical Activity, and Weight-Loss Intention," *Applied Economic Perspectives and Policy* 36, no. 1 (2013): 125–145.

9. Lili Wang, "Body Mass Index, Obesity, and Self-Control: A Comparison of Chronotypes," *Social Behavior & Personality* 24, no. 2 (1996): 313–320.

10. Alexandra A. Brewis, *Obesity: Cultural and Biocultural Perspectives* (New Brunswick, N.J.: Rutgers University Press, 2011), 117.

11. Ibid.

12. S. M. Phelan, D. J. Burgess, M. W. Yeazel, W. L. Hellerstedt, J. M. Griffin, and M. van Ryn, "Impact of Weight Bias and Stigma on Quality of Care and Outcomes for Patients with Obesity," *Obesity Reviews* 16, no. 4 (2015): 319–326.

13. K. Campbell, H. Engel, A. Timperio, C. Cooper, and D. Crawford, "Obesity Management: Australian General Practitioners' Attitudes and Practices," *Obesity Research* 8 (2000):

459–466; E. L. Harvey and A. J. Hill, "Health Professionals' Views of Overweight People and Smokers," *International Journal of Obesity and Related Metabolic Disorders* 25 (2001): 1253–1261; Y. Fogelman, S. Vinker, and J. Lachter, "Managing Obesity: A Survey of Attitudes and Practices among Young Israeli Primary Care Physicians," *International Journal of Obesity* 26 (2002): 1393–1397; A. Bocquier, P. Verger, A. Basdevant, et al., "Overweight and Obesity: Knowledge, Attitudes, and Practices of General Practitioners in France," *Obesity Research* 13 (2002): 787–795.

14. Kwan and Graves, *Framing Fat*, 37.

15. Regina G. Lawrence, "Framing Obesity: The Evolution of News Discourse on a Public Health Issue," *Press/Politics* 9, no. 3 (2004): 56–75; Sei-Hill Kim and L. Anne Willis, "Talking about Obesity: New Framing of Who Is Responsible for Causing and Fixing the Problem," *Journal of Health Communication* 12, no. 4 (2007): 359–376.

16. Joan Costa Font, Christina Hernandez-Quevedo, James Ted McDonald, James Ted, and Variyam N. Jayachandaran, "Understanding Healthy Lifestyles: The Role of Choice." *Applied Economic Perspectives and Policy* 35, no. 1 (2012): 1–6; Heidi Dressler, "Food Choice, Eating Behavior, and Food Liking Differs between Lean/Normal and Overweight/Obese Low Income Women," *Appetite* 65, no. 1 (2013): 145–152.

17. For one example, see S. A. Jebb and M. S. Moore, "Contribution of Sedentary Lifestyle and Inactivity to the Etiology of Overweight and Obesity: Current Evidence and Research Issues," *Medicine and Science in Sports Exercise* 31, no. 11 (1999): S534–S541.

18. Beatrice Thomas, "Fast Food, Late Nights to Blame for Obesity in Gulf-Top Doc," *Arabian Business*, October 5, 2013, www.arabianbusiness.com/fast-food-late-nights-blame-for -obesity-in-gulf-top-doc-521757.html.

19. Rob Stein, "US to Seek Changes to Major WHO Obesity Effort," *Boston Globe*, January 16, 2004, www.boston.com/news/nation/washington/articles/2004/01/16/us_to_seek _changes_to_major_who_obesity_effort/.

20. Michael Abramowitz, "Bush Urges Stepped-Up Campaign Against Childhood Obesity," *Washington Post*, February 2, 2007, www.washingtonpost.com/wpdyn/content/article /2007/02/01/AR2007020101701.html.

21. Carol L. Wilking and Richard A. Daynard, "Beyond Cheeseburgers: The Impact of Commonsense Consumption Acts on Obesity-Related Lawsuits," *Food and Drug Law Journal* 68, no. 3 (2013): 229–239.

22. Victoria Stagg Elliott, "States Battle Obesity Epidemic with New Laws," *American Medical News*, March 24, 2008, www.amednews.com/article/20080324/health/303249965/4/.

23. Ron Barnett, "S.C. Case Looks on Child Obesity as Child Abuse. But Is It?," *USA Today*, July 20, 2009, http://usatoday30.usatoday.com/news/health/weightloss/2009-07-20 -obesityboy_N.htm.

24. Owen Jacques, "Plan to Tax Fast Food and Promote Good Farming Hits Hurdle," *Central Queensland News*, February 4, 2014, www.cqnews.com.au/news/tax-fast-food-obesity -promote-healthy-farming/2159025/.

25. "Tonga Considers Beefed Up Anti-Fat Tax to Combat Obesity," ABC (Australian Broadcasting Commission), June 11, 2014, www.abc.net.au/news/2014-06-11/an-tonga -obesity/5514784.

26. Tara Lohan, "Japan Fines 'Fat People,' Companies Must Measure Waist Lines of Employees," Alternet.org, November 25, 2009, www.alternet.org/story/144185/japan_fines_ percent27fatpercent27_people,_companies_must_measure_waist_lines_of_employees.

27. "Gold for Gulf Dieters as Obesity Threatens $68bn Bill," *Arab News*, February 23, 2014, www.arabnews.com/news/529856.

28. Rebecca Smith, "Obesity Crisis: Get Paid to Lose Weight," *Telegraph*, January 24, 2008, www.telegraph.co.uk/news/uknews/1576430/Obesity-crisis-get-paid-to-lose-weight.html.

29. Embodying Bush's notion of personal responsibility, Oklahoma City mayor Mick Cornett, Indiana governor Mitch Daniels, and Arkansas governor Mike Huckabee all implemented campaigns to encourage diet and exercise among their respective state's citizens. Cornett challenged citizens of Oklahoma City to collectively lose one million pounds, with Cornett contributing forty of his own pounds toward the goal. The city also began investing more in pedestrian-friendly city infrastructure to encourage physical activity. Daniels's plan, "Ten in Ten," set a goal for each citizen to lose ten pounds in ten weeks. News spots for "Ten in Ten" depict Daniels running during his lunchtime workouts, while promotional materials for the initiative depict him exercising with an Indiana resident, Pam Smith, who is also a former contestant on *The Biggest Loser*. Even though Huckabee positions himself as an example of personal responsibility, himself losing around one hundred pounds, his "Healthy Arkansas" initiative focuses more on schools reporting BMI statistics to parents and "incentivizing" employees to take walking breaks or allowing them to turn unused sick days into vacation days. Similarly, Nashville encouraged its citizens to "Walk 100 Miles with the Mayor." Fort Worth, Texas, developed "FitWorth," which holds races and family fitness challenges, and Somerville, Massachusetts, now has the "Mayor's Fitness Challenge," which culminates in prizes and a citywide party.

30. Let's Move!, "Learn the Facts. Accomplishments" (2011), www.letsmove.gov.

31. Ben Brooks, "Obesity Cannot Be Controlled through Personal Responsibility Alone," *Guardian*, January 12, 2014, www.theguardian.com/commentisfree/2014/jan/13/obesity-cannot-be-controlled-through-personal-responsibility-alone.

32. Stuart Wolpert, "Dieting Does Not Work, UCLA Researchers Report," UCLA Newsroom, April 3, 2007, http://newsroom.ucla.edu/portal/ucla/dieting-does-not-work-ucla-researchers-7832.aspx.

33. Hillel Schwartz, *Never Satisfied: A Cultural History of Diets, Fantasies, and Fat* (New York: Free Press, 1986).

34. Gerald Walker, "The Great American Dieting Neurosis," *New York Times*, August 23, 1959.

35. Pat Lyons, "Prescription for Harm: Diet Industry Influence, Public Health Policy, and the "Obesity Epidemic," in *The Fat Studies Reader*, ed. Esther Rothblum and Sondra Solovay (New York: New York University Press, 2009), 75–85.

36. Anemona Hartocollis, "Diet Plan with Hormones Has Fans and Skeptics," *New York Times*, March 7, 2011, www.nytimes.com/2011/03/08/nyregion/08hcg.html?_r=1&ref=todayspaper.

37. Wolpert, "Dieting Does Not Work."

38. Alisha M. Wade, "Fatal Malnutrition 6 Years after Gastric Bypass Surgery," *Journal of the American Medical Association* 170, no. 11 (2010): 993.

39. For a more detailed history of the changing social and medical understandings of fat, see Peter N. Stearns, *Fat History: Bodies and Beauty in the Modern West* (New York: New York University Press, 2002); Amy Erdman Farrell, *Fat Shame: Stigma and the Fat Body in American Culture* (New York: New York University Press, 2011); Sander L. Gilman, *Fat: A Cultural History* (Malden, Mass.: Polity, 2013); Georges Vigarello and C. Jon Delogu, *The Metamorphoses of Fat: A History of Obesity* (New York: Columbia University Press, 2013).

40. For a more comprehensive overview of the history of medicalization, see David Armstrong, "Bodies of Knowledge/Knowledge of Bodies," in *Reassessing Foucault: Power, Medicine, and the Body*, ed. Colin Jones and Roy Porter (New York: Routledge, 1998) 17–27; Irving Zola, "Medicine as an Institution of Social Control," *Sociological Review* 20 (1972): 487–504; Ivan Illich, *Limits to Medicine—Medical Memesis: The Expropriation of Health* (Middlesex: Penguin, 1976).

41. Ray Moynihan and Alan Cassels, *Selling Sickness: How the World's Biggest Pharmaceutical Companies Are Turning Us All into Patients* (New York: Nation Books, 2005).

42. Saguy, *What's Wrong with Fat?*, 42.

43. American Society for Metabolic and Bariatric Surgery, "Estimate of Bariatric Surgery Numbers, 2011–2015" (July 2016), https://asmbs.org/resources/estimate-of-bariatric-surgery-numbers.

44. Andrew Pollack, "A.M.A. Recognizes Obesity as a Disease," *New York Times*, June 19, 2013, www.nytimes.com/2013/06/19/business/ama-recognizes-obesity-as-a-disease.html.

45. Kathleen LeBesco, "Fat Panic and the New Morality," in *Against Health: How Health Became the New Morality*, ed. Jonathan M. Metzl and Anna Kirkland (New York: New York University Press, 2010), 76.

46. Geri Aston, "Obesity as a Chronic Disease, Not a Character Flaw," *Hospitals and Health Networks Magazine*, January 11, 2017, www.hhnmag.com/articles/7901–obesity-as-a-chronic-disease-not-a-character-flaw.

47. Natalie C. Lippa and Saskia C. Sanderson, "Impact of Information about Obesity Genomics on the Stigmatization of Overweight Individuals: An Experimental Study," *Obesity* 20, no. 12 (2012): 2367–2376; S. Daníelsóttir, K. S. O'Brien, and A. Ciao, "Anti-fat Prejudice Reduction: A Review of Published Studies," *Obesity Facts* 3, no. 1 (2010): 47–58.

48. Geoffrey Kabat, "Why Labeling Obesity as a Disease Is a Big Mistake," *Forbes*, July 9, 2013, www.forbes.com/sites/geoffreykabat/2013/07/09/why-labeling-obesity-as-a-disease-is-a-big-mistake/#5dd82b3103b9.

49. Pollack, "A.M.A. Recognizes Obesity as a Disease."

50. Crystal Hoyt, Jeni Burnette, and Lisa Auster-Gussman, "Obesity Is a Disease: Examining the Self-Regulatory Impact of This Public-Health Message," *Psychological Science* 24, no. 4 (2014): 997–1002.

51. Annemarie Jutel, "Doctor's Orders: Diagnosis, Medical authority, and the Exploitation of the Fat Female Body," in *Biopolitics and the "Obesity Epidemic": Governing Bodies*, ed. Jan Wright and Valerie Harwood (New York: Routledge, 2009), 61–77.

52. Campos, *Obesity Myth*.

53. Gina Kolata, "Study Says Obesity Can Be Contagious," *New York Times*, July 25, 2007, www.nytimes.com/2007/07/25/health/25cnd-fat.html?_r=0.

54. Nicholas A. Christakis and James Fowler, "The Spread of Obesity in a Large Social Network over 32 Years," *New England Journal of Medicine* 357 (2007): 370–379.

55. Jim Landers, "Obesity Is Spreading Rapidly around the World," *Dallas News*, January 19, 2013, www.dallasnews.com/business/headlines/20130119–obesity-is-spreading-rapidly-around-world.ece.

56. K. Fujioka, "Follow-Up of Nutritional and Metabolic Problems after Bariatric Surgery," *Diabetes Care* 28, no. 2 (2005): 241–284.

57. D. O. Magro et al., "Long-Term Weight regain After Gastric Bypass: A 5-Year Prospective Study," *Obesity Surgery* 18, no. 6 (2008): 648–651; L. Davidson et al., "Resting Metabolic Rate and Fat Free Mass, Not Diet or Exercise, Predict Weight Regain 6 Years after Gastric Bypass Surgery," *Obesity* 20 (2012): S73–S74. Linda Bacon does an excellent job synthesizing research on bariatric surgery and provides a more exhaustive list of surgery complications, the heightened risks of mortality postsurgery, and concerns expressed by individuals within the medical field. See Linda Bacon, *Health at Every Size: The Surprising Truth about Your Weight* (Dallas: BenBella Books, 2008).

58. Michel Foucault, *Discipline and Punish: The Birth of Prison* (New York: Vintage, 1979).

59. Stuart Hall, "Introduction," in *Representation: Cultural Representations and Signifying Practices*, ed. Stuart Hall (London: Sage, 1997), 49.

60. Lauren Berlant, "Risky Bigness: On Obesity, Eating, and the Ambiguity of 'Health,'" in Metzl and Kirkland, *Against Health*, 26–39.

61. Foucault, *Discipline and Punish*.

62. For a thorough account of why contemporary society "fears" fat, see Susan Bordo, *Unbearable Weight* (Berkeley: University of California Press, 1993); Deborah Lupton, *Fat* (New York: Routledge, 2013).

63. Rebecca M. Puhl, Jamie Lee Peterson, Jenny A. DePierre, and Joerg Luedicke, "Headless, Hungry, and Unhealthy: A Video Content Analysis of Obese Person Portrayed in Online News," *Journal of Health Communication: International Perspectives* 18, no. 6 (2013): 686–702.

64. Deborah Morrison Thomson, "Big Food and the Body Politics of Personal Responsibility," *Southern Communication Journal* 74 (2009): 8.

65. J. Eric Oliver, *Fat Politics* (Oxford: Oxford University Press, 2006), 60.

66. Janna L. Fikkan and Esther Rothblum, "Is Fat a Feminist Issue? Exploring the Gendered Nature of Weight Bias," *Sex Roles* 66, nos. 9–10 (2011): 575–593.

67. Emily Ramshaw, "Victoria Hospital Won't Hire Very Obese Workers," *Texas Tribune*, March 26, 2012, www.texastribune.org/texas-health-resources/health-reform-and-texas/victoria-hospital-wont-hire-very-obese-workers/.

68. Joyce Huff, "Access to the Sky: Airplane Seats and Fat Bodies as Contested Spaces," in Rothblum and Solovay, *Fat Studies Reader*, 176–187.

69. Ashley Hetrick and Derek Attig, "Sitting Pretty: Fat Bodies, Classroom Desks, and Academic Excess," in Rothblum and Solovay, *Fat Studies Reader*, 197–204.

70. Tracy Royce, "The Shape of Abuse: Fat Oppression as a Form of Violence Against Women," in Rothblum and Solovay, *Fat Studies Reader*, 151–157.

71. Charisse W. Goodman, *The Invisible Woman: Confronting Weight Prejudice in America* (Carlsbad, Calif.: Gurze Books, 1995).

72. Rebecca M. Puhl, Tatiana Andreyeva, and Kelly D. Brownwell, "Perceptions of Weight Discrimination: Prevalence and Comparison to Race and Gender Discrimination in America," *International Journal of Obesity* 32, no. 6 (2008): 992–1000.

73. Anna MacDonald, "Study Finds Obese Women Experience Discrimination," ABC (Australia Broadcast Commission), May 1, 2012, www.abc.net.au/worldtoday/content/2012/s3492852.htm; Marla Dickerson and Meredith Mandell, "In Mexico, Young and Thin Are Often Job Requirements," *Los Angeles Times*, October 23, 2006, http://articles.latimes.com/2006/oct/23/business/fi-mexhiring23; Maureen Fan, "Chinese Women Sing to Fight Discrimination Against Obese," *Wenatchee World*, September 8, 2007, www.wenatcheeworld.com/news/2007/sep/08/chinese-women-sing-to-fight-discrimination/.

74. Dan Fletcher, "A Brief History of the Fat-Acceptance Movement," *Time*, July 31, 2009, http://content.time.com/time/nation/article/0,8599,1913858,00.html; Sondra Solovay and Esther Rothblum, "Introduction," in Rothblum and Solovay, *Fat Studies Reader*, 1–10.

75. Lupton, *Fat*, 67.

76. Paul Campos, "Our Absurd Fear of Fat," *New York Times*, January 2, 2013, www.nytimes.com/2013/01/03/opinion/our-imaginary-weight-problem.html; Nicholas D. Kristof, "Warnings from a Flabby Mouse," *New York Times*, January 19, 2013, www.nytimes.com/2013/01/20/opinion/sunday/kristof-warnings-from-a-flabby-mouse.html.

77. Laura Blue, "Being Overweight Is Linked to Lower Risk of Mortality," *Time*, January 2, 2013, http://healthland.time.com/2013/01/02/being-overweight-is-linked-to-lower-risk-of-mortality/.

78. Michelle Roberts, "People Can Be Fat yet Fit, Research Suggests," *BBC News Online*, September 4, 2012, www.bbc.co.uk/news/health-19474239.

79. Alessandra Stanley, "Women on TV Step Off the Scale," *New York Times*, October 11, 2012, www.nytimes.com/2012/10/14/arts/television/women-on-tv-step-off-the-scale.html ?pagewanted=1.

80. Farrell, *Fat Shame*, 14.

81. Shari Dworkin and Faye Linda Wachs, *Body Panic: Gender, Health, and the Selling of Fitness* (New York: New York University Press, 2009).

82. Kwan and Graves, *Framing Fat*, 37.

83. Michael Orr, "Plus-Size Barbie Sparks Online Debate over Body Image," *ABC News*, December 31, 2013, http://abcnews.go.com/blogs/headlines/2013/12/plus-size-barbie-sparks -online-debate-over-body-image/.

84. Abigail Jones, "The Fully Beauty Photo Project: Big Women Bare All," *Newsweek*, October 21, 2013, www.newsweek.com/full-beauty-photo-project-big-women-bare-all-636.

85. Blaize Stewart, "Issues with the Fat Acceptance Movement," *Odyssey*, August 12, 2014, www.theodysseyonline.com/issues-fat-acceptance-movement.

86. Christopher Friend, "Solve America's Obesity Problem with Shame," *Philly Mag*, October 22, 2012, www.phillymag.com/news/2012/10/12/solve-americas-obesity-problem -shame/.

87. Daniel J. Munoz, "Fat Acceptance Movement Utilizes Pseudoscience," *Daily Targum*, May 2, 2014, 9.

88. "Editorial: Fat Power Movement Dangerous," *Bayloriat*, May 2, 2014, http://baylorlariat .com/2014/05/02/editorial-fat-power-movement-dangerous/; Tammy Worth, "Is the Fat Acceptance Movement Bad for Our Health?," *CNN*, January 6, 2010, www.cnn.com/2010 /HEALTH/01/06/fat.acceptance/index.html.

89. Barbara Kay, "Fat Acceptance Is Not the Answer to Obesity," *National Post*, September 11, 2013.

90. Jennifer Lee, "A Big Fat Fight: The Case for Fat Activism," *Conversation*, June 22, 2012, http://theconversation.com/a-big-fat-fight-the-case-for-fat-activism-7743.

91. Dodi Stewart, "Happy Fat Acceptance Anniversary? 40 Years, Not Much Progress," *Jezebel*, July 31, 2009, http://jezebel.com/5327238/happy-fat-acceptance-anniversary-40-years -not-much-progress.

CHAPTER 3 — DOES TV MAKE YOU FAT?

1. Herbert Schiller, *Mass Communication and American Empire* (New York: Augustus M. Keeley, 1969); Walter Lippmann, "Television: Whose Creature? Whose Servant?," in *The Essential Lippmann: Political Philosophy for Liberal Democracy*, ed. Clinton Rossiter and James Lare (Cambridge, Mass.: Harvard University Press, 1982), 411–415; Nicholas Garnham, "Concepts of Culture: Public Policy and the Cultural Industries," *Cultural Studies* 1 (1987): 23–37.

2. Laurie Ouellette, *Viewers Like You? How Public TV Failed the People* (New York: Columbia University Press, 2002), 4.

3. J. Fred MacDonald, *Blacks and White TV: African Americans in Television since 1948* (Chicago: Nelson-Hall, 1992), xv.

4. Michael Curtin, *Redeeming the Wasteland: Television Documentary and Cold War Politics* (New Brunswick, N.J.: Rutgers University Press, 1995); MacDonald, *Blacks and White TV*.

5. Thomas Streeter, *Selling the Air: A Critique of the Policy of Commercial Broadcasting in the United States* (Chicago: University of Chicago Press, 1996), 189.

6. Anna McCarthy, *The Citizen Machine: Governing by Television in 1950s America* (New York: New Press, 2010).

7. Peter Miller and Nikolas Rose, *Governing the Present: Administering Economic, Social, and Personal Life* (Boston: Polity, 2008).

8. Laurie Ouellette and James Hay, "Makeover Television, Governmentality, and the Good Citizen," *Continuum* 22, no. 4 (2008): 471–484.

9. Chad Raphael, "The Political-Economic Origins of Reali-TV," in *Reality TV: Remaking Television Culture*, ed. Laurie Ouellette and Susan Murray (New York: New York University Press, 2004).

10. Nielson, "Americans Watching More TV Than Ever; Web and Mobile Video Up," Too" (May 20, 2009), http://blog.nielsen.com/nielsenwire/online_mobile/americans-watching -more-tv-than-ever/.

11. Brian Lowery, "Obesity and TV: Lift That Remote, and Bend and . . . ," *Broadcasting and Cable*, June 28, 2004.

12. "Round-the-Clock TV Rejected by Malaysia," *Toledo Blade*, August 17, 1995.

13. Paul Cullen, "One in Four Girls, One in Five Boys Now Overweight," *Irish Times*, March 15, 2007.

14. Terence Blacker, "Overweight, Overexposed, and Over Here," *Independent*, March 16, 2012.

15. Randy Shore, "Turn Off the TV to Fight the Fat, SFU Prof Urges; New Book Argues Panic over Child Obesity Masks Its Cause," *Vancouver Sun*, May 30, 2011.

16. Scott A. Lear et al., "The Association between Ownership of Common Household Devices and Obesity in High, Middle, and Low Income Countries," *Canadian Medical Association Journal* 186 (2014): 258–266.

17. Jill Pengelley, "TV Couch Potato Switches on to a Healthier Life," *Advertiser*, May 6, 2003.

18. J. Lakerveld et al., "Abdominal Obesity, TV Viewing Time, and Prospective Declines in Physical Activity," *Preventive Medicine* 53, nos. 4–5 (2011): 299–302.

19. Frank Hu, "Television Watching and Other Sedentary Behaviors in Relation to Risk of Obesity and Type 2 Diabetes Mellitus in Women," *Journal of the American Medical Association* 289, no. 14 (2012): 1785–1791.

20. Brad Dich, "Is Television Making You Fat?," *Broadcast Engineering*, December 2006.

21. S. L. Gortmaker et al., "Television Viewing as a Cause of Increasing Obesity among Children in the United States, 1986–1990," *Archives of Pediatrics and Adolescent Medicine* 150, no. 4 (1996): 356–363; R. E. Andersen et al., "Relationship of Physical Activity and Television Watching with Body Weight and Level of Fatness among Children," *Journal of the American Medical Association* 279 (1998): 938–942; B. Hernandez et al., "Association of Obesity with Physical Activity, Television Programs and Other Forms of Video Viewing among Children in Mexico City," *International Journal of Obesity* 23 (1999): 845–854; R. J. Hancox and R. Poulton, "Television Is Associated with Childhood Obesity: But Is It Clinically Important?," *International Journal of Obesity* 30 (2006): 171–175.

22. R. Boulos et al., "ObesiTV: How Television Is Influencing the Obesity Epidemic," *Physiology & Behavior* 107, no. 1 (2012): 146–153.

23. Ouellette, *Viewers Like You?*, 39.

24. Ibid., 33.

25. Robert McChesney, *Rich Media, Poor Democracy: Communication Politics in Dubious Times* (Urbana: University of Illinois Press, 1999), 200.

26. Drew Simshaw, "Survival of the Standard: Today's Public Interest Requirement in Television Broadcasting and the Return of Regulation," *Federal Communications Law Journal* 64, no. 2 (2012): 403.

27. Raymond Williams, *Television: Technology and Cultural Form* (New York: Routledge, 1974).

28. Ien Ang, *Desperately Seeking the Audience* (New York: Routledge, 1991), 103.

29. McChesney, *Rich Media, Poor Democracy*, 226.

30. Michael P. McCauley, "The Contested Meaning of Public Service in American Television," *Communication Review* 5 (2002): 229.

31. Douglas Kellner, "Public Access Television: Alternative Views," in *American Media and Mass Culture*, ed. Donald Lazere (Berkeley: University of California Press, 1987), 610.

32. Ibid.

33. Cited in Patricia Aufderheide, "Cable Television and the Public Interest," *Journal of Communication* 42, no. 1 (1991): 52–65.

34. Ibid., 53.

35. Simshaw, "Survival of the Standard," 407.

36. Ibid., 407.

37. Heather Hendershot, *Saturday Morning Censors: Television Regulation before the V-Chip* (Durham, N.C.: Duke University Press, 1999), 65.

38. Streeter, *Selling the Air*, 90.

39. Hendershot, *Saturday Morning Censors*, 5.

40. Bill McConnell, "Bloated Agenda: Critics Demand More Regulation, Even as the Industry Polices Itself," *Broadcasting and Cable*, June 14, 2004.

41. "Docs Want TV Fast-Food Ads Banned from Kids' Shows," *Huffington Post*, June 27, 2011, www.huffingtonpost.com/2011/06/27/doctors-ban-fast-foodads_n_885218.html.

42. E. Boyland et al., "Food Commercials Increase Preference for Energy-Dense Foods, Particularly in Children Who Watch More Television," *Pediatrics* 128, no. 1 (2011): e93–e100.

43. "TV Ads Lure Kids to Junk Food," *Straits Times*, June 30, 2011.

44. Bae Ji-Sook, "Junk Food Ads to Be Restricted," *Korea Times*, January 19, 2010.

45. "Study: Quebec Ban on Fast-Food Ads Reduced Consumption of Junk Food," *Medical Xpress*, January 2012, http://medicalxpress.com/news/2012-01-quebec-fast-food-ads-consumption-junk.html.

46. World Health Organization, "Global Strategy on Diet, Physical Activity and Health" (Report WHA57.17 2004), www.who.int/gb/ebwha/pdf_files/WHA57/A57_R17-en.pdf.

47. "Fat TV Ad Ban Plan," *Sunday Mercury*, March 18, 2012.

48. Mark Sweney, "Total Ban for Junk Food Ads around Kids' Shows," *Guardian*, November 17, 2006, www.guardian.co.uk/society/2006/nov/17/health.food.

49. Nema-Tamara Patel and Tom Farmery, "Childhood Obesity in England: See How Your Area Compares," *Guardian*, December 19, 2011, www.guardian.co.uk/news/datablog/2011/dec/19/obesity-childhood-statistics.

50. Corinna Hawkes, "Marketing Food to Children: The Global Regulatory Environment" (Geneva: World Health Organization, 2004), http://whqlibdoc.who.int/publications/2004/9241591579.pdf.

51. Ibid.

52. Jane Martin and Boyd, "Junk Logic Is Shielding Junk Food Adverts," *Age*, September 2, 2009.

53. Ira Teinowitz, "Bush Nominates Tate to Full FCC Term," *Television Week* 26, nos. 26/27 (2007).

54. John Eggerton, "Kid-Obesity Report Due to Congress in July," *Broadcasting and Cable*, March 26, 2007.

55. "TV's Duty to Kids," *Broadcasting and Cable,* March 30, 2007, www.broadcastingcable.com/news/news-articles/tvs-duty-kids/82269; John Eggerton, "Where's the Beef?" *Broadcasting and Cable,* December 17, 2007.

56. Sam Hananel, "FCC to Study Ads, Kids' Weight for Link," *The Washington Post,* September 27, 2006, *http://www.washingtonpost.com/wp-dyn/content/article/2006/09/27/AR2006092701539.html.*

57. Diane Aden Hayes, "The Children's Hour Revisited: The Children's Television Act of 1990," *Federal Communications Law Journal* 46, no. 2 (1994): Article 5.

58. Todd Shields, "FCC Fines Viacom, ABC Family over Kids' Ads Rules," *Ad Week,* October 21, 2004.

59. Nat Ives, "The Media Business: Advertising; As National Geographic Explores Obesity, Critics Question the Food Ads in Its Children's Magazine," *New York Times,* July 21, 2004.

60. Hendershot, *Saturday Morning Censors,* 18.

61. McCarthy, *Citizen Machine,* 24.

62. Ibid., 27.

63. Anooska Tucker-Evans, "Obesity Rules TV—Loser Shows Are a Winner," *Sunday Mail,* March 28, 2010.

64. Michael Schneider, "Reality TV Continues Fascination with Fat," *Variety,* July 25, 2009.

65. Michael Schneider, "Networks Living in a FAT City," *Variety,* July 27–August 2, 2009.

66. "Weight Loss TV Show Draws Viewers in India," *Bangladesh News,* June 8, 2007.

67. Rafel Romo, "Mexico's Other Enemy: Obesity Rates Triple in Last Three Decades," *CNN World,* January 4, 2011, http://articles.cnn.com/20110104/world/mexico.obesity_1_obesity-rates-obese-people-junk-food?_s=PM:WORLD.

68. Akiela Hope, "Caribbean Obesity Rates Get Wider," *Guardian,* July 25, 2010, http://test.guardian.co.tt/index.php?q=features/life/2010/07/25/caribbean-obesity-rates-get-wider-hf.

69. "Kenya's Growing Middle Class," *New Zealand Herald,* August 10, 2012, www.nzherald.co.nz/business/news/article.cfm?c_id=3&objectid=10825807.

70. Philip Boffey, "What if It Weren't Called Pink Slime? . . . ," *New York Times,* May 13, 2012; David Robertson, "It Began as a Battle of Childhood Obesity, but Middle America Is Fighting to Defend Its 'Pink Slime,'" *Times,* March 31, 2012.

71. Brian Lowery, "Review: 'The Weight of the Nation," *Variety,* May 13, 2012, https://variety.com/2012/tv/reviews/the-weight-of-the-nation-1117947544/.

72. Gary Taubes, "The New Obesity Campaigns Have It All Wrong," *Newsweek,* May 24, 2012.

73. Curtin, *Redeeming the Wasteland,* 3.

74. These workouts basically detail exercise routines that can be performed from the comfort of one's own couch while watching television or during commercial breaks.

75. Ian Burrell, "BBC's Fat Nation Strives to Save Britain from Obesity," *Independent,* July 28, 2004.

76. U.S. Department of Health and Human Services, Office of Minority Health, "Obesity and African Americans," http://minorityhealth.hhs.gov/templates/content.aspx?ID=6456.

77. "The BET Foundation Tackles Obesity Head On with Its Fourth Annual 'A Healthy Bet' Fitness Challenge," *PR Newswire,* 2007, www.prnewswire.com/news-releases/the-bet-foundation-tackles-obesity-head-on-with-its-fourth-annual-a-healthy-bet-fitness-challenge-54993567.html.

78. Centers for Disease Control and Prevention, "BET Foundation Awards Presented at CDC" (2009), www.cdc.gov/partners/Archive/BET_Foundation/index.html.

79. "BET Foundation and General Mills Launch Comprehensive Healthy Living ('A Healthy BET') to Fight Obesity among African Americans," *PR Newswire*, 2003, www .prnewswire.com/news-releases-test/bet-foundation-and-general-mills-launch -comprehensive-healthy-living-program-a-healthy-bet-to-fight-obesity-among-african -americans-59030537.html.

80. James Annesi and Gorjala Srinivasa, "Body Satisfaction and Overall Mood: Effects of Race on Exercises of Obesity," *Social Behavior and Personality* 38, no. 8 (2010): 1105–1109.

81. Kathleen LeBesco, *Revolting Bodies: The Struggle to Redefine Fat Identity* (Amherst: University of Massachusetts Press, 2004), 31.

82. Ibid.

83. Patricia Hill Collins, *Black Feminist Thought: Knowledge, Consciousness and the Politics of Empowerment*, 2nd ed. (London: HarperCollins, 2000); Melissa A. Milkie, "Social Comparisons, Reflected Appraisals, and Mass Media: The Impact of Pervasive Beauty Images on Black and White Girls' Self-Concepts," *Social Psychology Quarterly* 62, no. 2 (1999): 190–210; Andria M. Thomas et al., "Perceptions of Obesity: Black and White Differences," *Journal of Cultural Diversity* 15, no. 4 (2008): 174–180.

84. Andrea Elizabeth Shaw, *The Embodiment of Disobedience: Fat Black Women's Unruly Political Bodies* (Lanham, Md.: Lexington Books, 2006), 6–9.

85. Katherine Sender and Margaret Sullivan, "Epidemics of Will, Failures of Self-Esteem: Responding to Fat Bodies in *The Biggest Loser* and *What Not to Wear*," *Continuum* 22, no. 4 (2008): 573–584.

86. Abigail Saguy, *What's Wrong with Fat?* (Oxford: Oxford University Press, 2013), 78.

87. D. Schooler et al., "Who's That Girl: Television's Role in the Body Image Development of Young White and Black Women," *Psychology of Women Quarterly* 28 (2004): 38–47.

88. M. Lovejoy, "Disturbances in the Social Body: Differences in Body Image and Eating Problems among African American and White Women," *Gender & Society* 15 (2001): 239–261.

89. Natalie Barturka, Paige P. Hornsby, and John B. Schorling, "Clinical Implications of Body Image among Rural African-American Women," *Journal of General Internal Medicine* 15, no. 4 (2000): 235–241.

90. S. Caprio et al., "Influence of Race, Ethnicity, and Culture on Childhood Obesity: Implications for Prevention and Treatment. A Consensus Statement of Shaping America's Health and the Obesity Society," *Diabetes Care* 31, no. 11 (2008): 2211–2221.

91. V. J. Rideout and E. Hamel, *The Media Family: Electronic Media in the Lives of Infants, Toddlers, and Preschoolers, and Their Parents* (Menlo Park, Calif.: Kaiser Family Foundation, 2006).

92. Alexandra A. Brewis, *Obesity: Cultural and Biocultural Perspectives* (New Brunswick, N.J.: Rutgers University Press, 2011), 77.

93. Saguy, *What's Wrong with Fat?*, 19.

94. Ibid., 97.

95. Deborah Lupton, *Fat* (New York: Routledge, 2013), 47.

96. Shaw, *Embodiment of Disobedience*, 9.

97. Hendershot, *Saturday Morning Censors*, 3.

98. James E. Brody, "Personal Health; TV's Tool on Young Minds and Bodies," *New York Times*, August 3, 2004.

99. "Children Are TV-Tubbies," *Daily Telegraph*, January 23, 2002.

100. A. Heilmann, P. Rouxel, E. Fitzsimmons, Y. Kelly, and R.G. Watt, "Longitudinal Associations Between Television in the Bedroom and Body Fatness in a U.K. Cohort Study," *International Journal of Obesity* 41 (2017): 1503–1509.

101. Julian Armstrong, "Diets Not Working, Kids Glue to Tube, Conference Told," *Star Phoenix*, June 17, 2006.

102. Sue Hubbard, "TV Link; Cut Child's Screen Time to Boost Health," *Vancouver Province*, July 10, 2011.

103. Hendershot, *Saturday Morning Censors*, 24.

104. Ibid., 22.

105. Laura Dawes, *Childhood Obesity in America: Biography of an Epidemic* (Cambridge, Mass.: Harvard University Press, 2014), 184.

106. Bill McConnell, "One Fat Target: How Much Longer Can TV Gorge Itself on Children's Advertising?," *Broadcasting and Cable*, March 8, 2004.

107. Ibid.

108. McConnell, "Bloated Agenda."

109. Lisa Haugsted, "Nick Goes Out to 'Play,'" *Multichannel News*, September 24, 2007.

110. McConnell, "One Fat Target."

111. Ibid.

112. Ibid.

113. Maline Saval, "A Wealth of Health in Net's Social Effects," *Variety*, October 1–7, 2012.

114. Jacob Bauder, "TV Shows Help Get Preschoolers Moving," *Times Daily*, December 16, 2004.

115. Mimi Turner, "'Lazytown' Founder Sells to Turner Broadcasting for $25 Million," *Hollywood Reporter*, September 8, 2011, www.hollywoodreporter.com/news/lazytown-founder-sells-turner-broadcasting-232908.

116. Janice Burns, "Kids Toon in to Keep Fit; New TV 'Toddlerobics,'" *Daily Record*, November 2, 2007.

117. Catherine Dawson, "Can TV Help Your Kids Get Fit?," *Globe and Mail*, April 3, 2009, http://m.theglobeandmail.com/life/can-tv-help-your-kids-get-fit/article794613.

118. Katherine Rushton, "'Bo on the Go!' Lands Six Deals," *Broadcast Magazine*, September 3, 2008.

119. Gretchen Reynolds, "Don't Just Sit There," *New York Times*, April 28, 2012, www.nytimes.com/2012/04/29/sunday-review/stand-up-for-fitness.html.

120. "Battling the Obesity Crisis with a Ravenous Blue Monster and Singing Vegetables" (Sesame Street Healthy Habits for Life Initiative, 2012), www.sesameworkshop.org/what-we-do/our-initiatives/healthy-habits-for-life.html?o=88&c=category.

121. Tom Fitzsimmons, "TV Channel Tells Kids to Get Outside," *Dominion Post*, November 29, 2007.

122. Austin Fenner, "Kraft Junking Toon-Time Ads. Food Giant Gets the Guilties over Kids' Bad Diets," *New York Daily News*, January 13, 2005.

123. Edmund Lee and Kate Andersen Bower, "Disney Will Ban Junk Food Ads on Kids Programming by 2015," *Bloomberg Businessweek*, June 5, 2012, www.businessweek.com/news/2012-06-05/disney-to-impose-new-rules-on-junk-food-ads-on-kid-s-shows.

124. These standards are the nutritional equivalent to eating half of a Snickers candy bar.

125. Dawn Chmielewski, "Disney Bans Junk Food Advertising on Programs for Children," *Los Angeles Times*, June 6, 2012, http://articles.latimes.com/2012/jun/06/business/la-fi-ct-disney-food-ads-20120606.

126. Nicola Stow, "Stop TV Junk Food Ads for Children Says EU," *Evening News*, January 20, 2005.

127. Eggerton, "Kid-Obesity Report."

CHAPTER 4 — THE GLOBESITY EPIDEMIC

1. D. L. Christensen, "Obesity and Regional Fat Distribution in Kenyan Populations: Impact of Ethnicity and Urbanization," *Annals of Human Biology* 35, no. 2 (2008): 232–249.

2. Nanci Hellmich, "Obesity Conference Takes on Weight of the World," *USA Today*, September 1, 1998.

3. Lauren Berlant, *Cruel Optimism* (Durham, N.C.: Duke University Press, 2007).

4. Ian Birrell, "Obesity: Africa's New Crisis," *Guardian*, September 21, 2014, www.theguardian .com/society/2014/sep/21/obesity-africas-new-crisis.

5. Tasha Oren, "Reiterational Texts and Global Imagination: Television Strikes Back," in *Global Television Formats: Understanding Television Across Borders,* eds. Tasha Oren and Sharon Shahaf (New York: Routledge), 374.

6. Jonathan Bignell, *Big Brother: Reality TV in the Twenty-First Century* (Basingstoke: Palgrave Macmillan, 2005), 40.

7. Tania Lewis, "Changing Rooms, Biggest Losers, and Backyard Blitzes: A History of Makeover Television in the United Kingdom, United States, and Australia," in *TV Transformations: Revealing the Makeover Show,* ed. Tania Lewis (New York: Routledge, 2009), 16.

8. Jeffrey O. Valisno, "Everyone Wants to Be the 'Biggest Loser,'" *Business World*, November 24, 2009.

9. Ibid.

10. Sharlene Nagy Hesse-Biber, *The Cult of Thinness* (Oxford: Oxford University Press, 2006).

11. Abigail Saguy, *What's Wrong with Fat?* (Oxford: Oxford University Press, 2013).

12. Nanci Hellmich, "Panel: Obesity Is Century's Greatest Public Health Threat," *USA Today*, June 15, 2010, http://usatoday30.usatoday.com/news/health/weightloss/2010-06-15 -dietaryguidelines16_ST_N.htm.

13. Sarah West, "Obesity: A Threat to Global Health" (World Cancer Research Fund, December 14, 2012), www.wcrf.org/blog/obesity-a-threat-to-global-health/.

14. Alexandra Sifferlin, "Weight of the World: Globally, Adults Are 16.5 Million Tons Overweight," *Time*, June 12, 2018, http://healthland.time.com/2012/06/18/weight-of-the-world -globally-adults-are-overweight-by-16-5-million-tons/.

15. Eric J. Oliver and T. Lee, "Public Opinion and the Politics of Obesity," *Journal of Health Politics, Policy, and Law* 30, no. 5 (2005): 923–954.

16. Scott Conroy, "Obesity an 'International Scourge,'" *CBS News*, September 3, 2006, www.cbsnews.com/news/obesity-an-international-scourge/.

17. World Health Organization, "Obesity Situation and Trends" (2008), www.who.int /gho/ncd/risk_factors/overweight/en/index.html.

18. World Health Organization, "World Health Statistics 2006," www.who.int/whosis /whostat2006/en/index.html.

19. Mike Desmond, "Obesity Expert Says World Is Picking Up America's 'Bad Habits,'" WBFO 88.7, October 17, 2013, http://news.wbfo.org/post/obesity-expert-says-world-picking -americas-bad-habits.

20. Mohammed Alkhereiji, "Fighting the Saudi Battle of the Bulge," *Arab News*, March 19, 2002, www.arabnews.com/node/219264.

21. Oliver Williams, "America's Deadliest Export," *New Internationalist*, August 22, 2014, https://newint.org/blog/2014/08/22/america-obesity-export.

22. Harold Maass, "Is Obesity America's Most Influential Export," *Week*, September 6, 2013, http://theweek.com/articles/460312/obesity-americas-most-influential-export.

23. Matthew Mientka, "America Exports Obesity around the World, as Developing World Sees Health Crisis," *Medical Daily*, September 7, 2013, www.medicaldaily.com/america -exports-obesity-around-world-developing-world-sees-health-crisis-255941.

24. Leah Schmidt, "Qatar Is the World's Wealthiest Country, but Also among Most Obese," *Mic*, March 9, 2012, https://mic.com/articles/5155/qatar-is-world-s-wealthiest-country-but -also-among-most-obese#.jrZHKqbN6.

25. Sarah E. Clark et al., "Exporting Obesity: US Farm and Trade Policy and the Transformation of the Mexican Consumer Food Environment," *International Journal of Occupational and Environmental Health* 18, no. 1 (2012): 53–64.

26. John Norris, "How America Is Exporting Its Obesity Epidemic," *Denver Post*, September 9, 2013, www.denverpost.com/2013/09/09/how-america-is-exporting-its-obesity-epidemic/.

27. Saguy, *What's Wrong with Fat?*, 47.

28. Ibid.

29. Katherine Flegal et al., "Aim for Healthy Weight: What Is the Target?," *Journal of Nutrition* 131 (2001): 440S–450S.

30. J. Eric Oliver, *Fat Politics* (Oxford: Oxford University Press, 2006), 40.

31. Laura Jennings, "Public Fat: Canadian Provincial Government and Fat on the Web," in *The Fat Studies Reader*, ed. Esther Rothblum and Sondra Solovay (New York: New York University Press, 2009), 88.

32. "Who's Fat? New Definition Adopted," *CNN*, June 17, 1998, www.cnn.com/HEALTH /9806/17/weight.guidelines/.

33. Ibid.

34. Lauren Berlant argues in *Cruel Optimism* that the labeling of AIDS as an epidemic revealed the term to be part of an argument about classification, casualty, etc. rather than a neutral description.

35. Mercedes de Onis et al., "Worldwide Implementation of the WHO Child Growth Standards," *Public Health Nutrition* 15 (2012): 1603–1610.

36. Christine Halse, "Bio-Citizenship: Virtue Discourses and the Birth of the Bio-Citizen," *Biopolitics and the 'Obesity Epidemic': Governing Bodies* (New York: Routledge, 2012), 55.

37. Nikolas Rose, "Medicine, History, and the Present," in *Reassessing Foucault: Power, Medicine, and the Body*, ed. Colin Jones and Roy Porter (New York: Routledge, 1998), 37.

38. Kirsten Ostherr, "Invisible Invaders: The Global Body in Public Health Frames," in *Cultural Sutures: Medicine and Medicine*, ed. Lester D. Friedman (Durham, N.C.: Duke University Press, 2004), 300–302.

39. Emma Rich and John Evans, "Performative Health in Schools: Welfare Policy, Neoliberalism, and Social Regulation," in *Biopolitics and the "Obesity Epidemic": Governing Bodies*, ed. Jan Wright and Valerie Harwood (New York: Routledge, 2009), 163.

40. Alexandra A. Brewis et al., "Body Norms and Fat Stigma in Global Perspective," *Current Anthropology* 52, no. 2 (2011): 269–276.

41. Ibid., 274.

42. Denise Ryan, "Fat Prejudice on the Rise," *Calgary Herald*, April 4, 2011.

43. Jina H. Yoo, "No Clear Winner: Effects of *The Biggest Loser* on the Stigmatization of Obese Persons," *Health Communication*, 28, no. 3 (2013): 294–303.

44. Timothy Havens, *Global Television Marketplace* (London: British Film Institute, 2006), 3.

45. Giampierto Gobo, "Glocalizing Methodology? The Encounter between Local Methodologies," *International Journal of Social Research Methodology* 14, no. 6 (2011): 428.

46. Albert Moran, *Copycat TV: Globalisation, Program Formats, and Cultural Identity* (Bedfordshire: University of Luton Press, 1998), 13.

47. Silvio Waisbord, "McTV: Understanding the Global Popularity of Television Formats," in *Television: The Critical View*, 7th ed., ed. Horace Newcomb (Oxford: Oxford University Press, 2007), 360.

48. Moran, *Copycat TV*, 294.

49. Caryn James, "Gaunt to Gargantuan and Back: The Atkins Method of Acting," *New York Times*, October 26, 2004, www.nytimes.com/2004/10/26/movies/gaunt-to-gargantuan-and-back-the-atkins-method-of-acting.html?mcubz=3&_r=0; Gillian Flynn, "The Biggest Loser," *Entertainment Weekly*, December 4, 2004, http://ew.com/article/2004/12/14/biggest-loser/.

50. Jonathan Bignell, *Big Brother: Reality TV in the Twenty-First Century* (United Kingdom: Palgrave Macmillan, 2005), 40.

51. A. J. Marechal, "Integration Partners Key as 'Biggest Loser' Returns," *Variety*, January 7, 2013, http://variety.com/2013/tv/news/integration-partners-key-as-biggest-loser-returns-1118064236/.

52. Gail Schiller, "'Loser' Gains with Brand Expansion," *Hollywood Reporter*, October 3, 2007, www.hollywoodreporter.com/news/loser-gains-brand-expansion-151541.

53. The WHO views a DALY as one year of "healthy" life lost due to disability and/or disease.

54. "Big Tent to Rep *Biggest Loser*," *License Mag*, October 22, 2013, www.licensemag.com/license-global/big-tent-rep-biggest-loser.

55. Katherine Sender and Margaret Sullivan, "Epidemics of Will, Failures of Self-Esteem: Responding to Fat Bodies in *The Biggest Loser* and *What Not to Wear*," in Lewis, *TV Transformations*, 139.

56. Lewis, "Changing Rooms, Biggest Losers, and Backyard Blitzes," 16.

57. Mimi Turner, "ITV Takes a Shine to 'Biggest Loser,'" *Hollywood Reporter*, November 13, 2008, www.hollywoodreporter.com/news/itv-takes-a-shine-biggest-122924.

58. Tania Lewis, "From Global to Glocal: Australianizing the Makeover Format," *TV Formats Worldwide: Localizing Global Programs*, ed. Albert Moran (Chicago: University of Chicago Press, 2009).

59. Ibid., 304.

60. Sarrah Le Marquand, "Losing It—The Power Struggles, Mind Games and Personal Victories behind *The Biggest Loser*—The Losing Battle," *Daily Telegraph* (Sydney), April 26, 2006.

61. Phillip Koch, "Weighty Winners; Readers Vote *The Biggest Loser* Our Most Stupid Show," *Sunday Herald Sun* (Melbourne), April 2, 2006.

62. Annalise Walker, "Unrealistic and Cruel, Say Experts; *Biggest Loser* Just 'A Big Turn-Off'," *Sunday Herald Sun* (Melbourne), February19, 2006.

63. Alex Murdoch, "Escapism on TV a Reality Lesson," *Courier Mail* (Brisbane), July 1, 2006.

64. Koch, "Weighty Winners."

65. Geoff Shearer, "Big Share in Weight Loss Show," *Courier Mail* (Brisbane), January 22, 2010.

66. Programs normally rationalize the exhibition of large bodies in one of two ways. First, extremely large participants demonstrate to viewers at home that if someone of such a large size can exercise to lose weight, viewers can too. Second, those individuals are framed as being in need of the most help or as being close to death due to their sizes. Extremely

large bodies also add drama to transformations, which is undoubtedly believed by producers to be good for ratings.

67. "Fresh Start for Kinder Loser," *Sydney Morning Herald*, March 20, 2017.

68. "Major Makeover for *The Biggest Loser*," *Coffs Coast Advocate*, March 8, 2017.

69. Ibid.

70. Lindsay Wise, "Whose Reality is Real? Ethical Reality TV Trends Offers 'Culturally Authentic' Alternative to Western Formats," in *The Real (Arab) World: Is Reality TV Democratizing the Middle East?* (Cairo: American University of Cairo Press, 2005), 49, emphasis added.

71. Nourah Almaiman, "Loser Becomes Winner: Translating Reality Shows for the Arab World" (American University of Sharjah, 2012), 47.

72. IPROD, "The Biggest Loser," www.iprod.tv/reality-the-biggest-loser.html.

73. Almaiman, "Loser Becomes Winner," 50–51.

74. Sara Yin, "Hard Act to Swallow; It's a Challenge for Networks to Adapt Western Reality TV Shows for Asian Tastes," *South China Morning Post*, September 22, 2009.

75. Boon Chan, "Asian Spin-Offs Win; With Slight Tweaks, Asian Versions of Reality Shows Gain More Viewers, Mileage and Sponsorship Here," *Straits Times* (Singapore), October 16, 2009.

76. Valisno, "Everyone Wants to Be the 'Biggest Loser.'"

77. Yin, "Hard Act to Swallow."

78. "Losing Big Wins Ratings; *The Biggest Loser Asia*," *Television Asia* 17, no. 3 (2010): 44.

79. Frankie Chee, "Counting Those Calories; Combining a Proper Diet with Exercise Is the Key to Effective Weight Loss," *Straits Times* (Singapore), October 2, 2010.

80. Chan, "Asian Spin-Offs Win."

81. Jeffrey O. Valisno, "Hallmarks Weight-Loss Show First Attempt at Asian Production," *Business World*, July 21, 2009.

82. S. Indramalar, "Want to Be a Big Loser?," *Star*, July 31, 2009, www.thestar.com.my /lifestyle/entertainment/tv/news/2009/07/31/want-to-be-a-big-loser/.

83. Valisno, "Everyone Wants to Be the 'Biggest Loser.'"

84. Dennis Chua, "Taking Charge of Their Lives by 'Losing Big,'" *New Straits Times* (Malaysia), June 14, 2010.

85. Yip Wai Yee and Natasha Ann Zachariah, "*Biggest Loser* Too Much?; Doctors Say Losing Weight Too Fast, Such as What *Biggest Loser* Winner Deveraj Did, Can Lead to Health Complications," *Straits Times* (Singapore), December 16, 2010.

86. Noel Chelliah, "*The Biggest Loser Asia*—Asia's Biggest Disappointment to the Fitness Industry," *Daily Muscle*, January 14, 2010, www.dailymuscle.com/2010/01/14/the-biggest -loser-asia-asias-biggest-dissapointment-to-the-fitness-industry/.

87. Ibid.

88. Chan, "Asian Spin-Offs Win."

89. "The Ministry to Decide on Reality Television Shows," *Star* (Malaysia), September 23, 2005.

90. "Reality Shows to Be Vetted for Negative Effects," *Star* (Malaysia), June 27, 2006, www .thestar.com.my/news/nation/2006/06/27/reality-shows-to-be-vetted-for-negative-effects/.

91. Diana Tjoa et al., "Reality TV in Asia: Indonesia, Malaysia, & Taiwan," May–June 2011, https://realitytvinasia.wordpress.com/.

92. Nancy Pollock, "Social Fattening Patterns in the Pacific: The Positive Side of Obesity—A Naru Case Study," in *Social Aspects of Obesity: Culture and Ecology of Food and Nutrition*, ed.

Igor De Garine and Nancy J. Pollock (New York: Taylor & Francis, 1995), 88; Jaehee Jung and Gordon B. Forbes, "Body Dissatisfaction and Disordered Eating: The Glocalization of Western Appearance Ideals," in *Feminist and Women's Rights Worldwide*, vol. 1, ed. Michele Antoinette Paludi (Westport, Conn.: Praeger, 2009), 177.

93. Lynn L. Farrales and Gwen E. Chapman, "Filipino Women Living in Canada: Constructing Meanings of Body, Food, and Health," *Health Care for Women International* 20, no. 2 (1999): 179–194. Although, contrary to these assumptions, some young women detail the ways in which Filipino culture is body shaming (given the social norm to comment on other people's appearance) and argue there is instead a preference for thinness, which could be an example of shifting norms or of limitations to the types of "fat" that are deemed desirable. For examples, please see Erica Waters, "Let's Talk about Body Shaming in the Philippines," *Nextshark*, May 19, 2017, https://nextshark.com/lets-talk-body-shaming-philippines/; Nina Penalosa, "When Bullying Follows You Home: Growing Up Chubby and Filipino," *Yourvoicemag*, March 23, 2016, https://wearyourvoicemag.com/body-politics/growing-up-chubby-and-filipino.

94. "Pacific Islanders Pay Heavy Price for Abandoning Traditional Diet," *Bulletin of the World Health Organization* 88, no. 7 (2010): 481–560, www.who.int/bulletin/volumes/88/7/10-010710/en/.

95. "Sharon Cuneta Tackles Obesity in 'Bignating Pinoy: The Biggest Loser Primer,'" *Starmometer*, May 13, 2011, www.starmometer.com/2011/05/13/sharon-cuneta-tackles-obesity-in-bigating-pinoy-the-biggest-loser-primer/.

96. "Press Statement from ABS-CBN," Philippine Entertainment Portal, May 27, 2011, www.pep.ph/guide/tv/8223/sharon-cuneta-encourages-everyone-to-embrace-a-healthy-lifestyle/1/2#focus.

97. Gretchen A. Stevens et al., "National, Regional, and Global Trends in Adult Overweight and Obesity Prevalences," *Popular Health Metrics* 10, no. 1 (2012): 22.

98. Ien Ang, "Culture and Communication: Towards an Ethnographic Critique of Media Consumption in the Transnational Media System," *European Journal of Communication* 5 (1990): 252–255.

99. Andrea Crossan, "In Kenya's Version of 'The Biggest Loser,' Contestants Win for Healthy Living, Not Just Dropping Pounds," KUOW 94.9, December 17, 2015, http://kuow.org/post/kenyas-version-biggest-loser-contestants-win-healthy-living-not-just-dropping-pounds.

100. Ibid.

101. Ibid.

102. Libby Coleman, "Kenya's 'Biggest Loser'—But with Dancing," *OZY*, January 10, 2017, www.ozy.com/good-sht/kenyas-biggest-loser-but-with-dancing/67135.

103. Moran, *Copycat TV*, cited in Lewis, "From Global to Glocal," 304

104. Dana Heller, "Intelligent Self-Design," *Television and New Media* 10, no. 1 (2009): 78.

105. Aaron Barnhart, "'Biggest Loser,' Other Reality Shows Find Success with Small Budget, Strong Personalities," *Pop Matters*, December 17, 2010, www.popmatters.com/article/134955–biggest-loser-other-reality-shows/.

106. Ibid.

CHAPTER 5 —— EXERCISING CONTROL AND THE ILLOGICS OF
WEIGHT-LOSS TELEVISION

1. Andrew Hampp, "Controversy Can't Slow 'Biggest Loser,'" *Advertising Age* 81, no. 27 (2010): 12.

2. Tom Huddleston Jr., "NBC Under Pressure to Cancel 'The Biggest Loser,'" *Fortune*, May 23, 2016, http://fortune.com/2016/05/23/biggest-loser-nbc-contestants/.

3. Edward Wyatt, "On 'The Biggest Loser,' Health Can Take a Back Seat," *New York Times*, November 24, 2009, www.nytimes.com/2009/11/25/business/media/25loser.html?mtrref =undefined.

4. James Fell, "'It's a Miracle No One Has Died Yet': *The Biggest Loser* Returns, Despite Critics' Warnings," *Guardian*, January 4, 2016, www.theguardian.com/tv-and-radio/2016 /jan/04/the-biggest-loser-returns-despite-critics-warnings.

5. Ibid.

6. Robert Thompson, "Finding Happiness between Commercials," *Chronicle of Higher Education* 17 (2003): B4, cited in Dana Heller, "Before: 'Things Just Keep Getting Better . . . ,'" in *The Great American Makeover: Television, History, and Nation*, ed. Dana Heller (New York: Palgrave Macmillan, 2006), 2.

7. Marsha F. Cassidy, "The Cinderella Makeover: *Glamour Girl*, Television Misery Shows, and 1950s Femininity," in Heller, *Great American Makeover*, 125–139.

8. Amber Watts, "*Queen for a Day*: Remaking Consumer Culture, One Woman at a Time," in Heller, *Great American Makeover*, 141–158.

9. Tania Lewis, ed., *TV Transformations: Revealing the Makeover Show* (New York: Routledge, 2013),13–14.

10. Dana Heller, *Makeover Television: Realities Remolded* (New York: I.B. Tauris, 2007).

11. Laurie Ouellette and James Hay, "Makeover Television, Governmentality, and the Good Citizen," *Continuum* 22, no. 4 (2008): 471–484.

12. Ibid., 476.

13. Amanda Hall Gallagher and Lisa Pecot-Hébert, "You Need a Makeover!": The Social Construction of Female Body Image in *A Makeover Story, What Not to Wear*, and *Extreme Makeover*," *Popular Communication* 5, no. 1 (2007): 58–63.

14. Michael Silk, Jessica Francombe, and F. Bachelor, "*The Biggest Loser*: The Discursive Constitution of Fatness," *Interactions: Studies in Communication and Culture* 1, no. 3 (2009): 370.

15. Ouellette and Hay, "Makeover Television."

16. Megan Warin, *Abject Relations: Everyday Worlds of Anorexia* (New Brunswick, N.J.: Rutgers University Press, 2009); Julie Ferris and Karen Pitcher, "Objectify(ing) the Abject: The Excessive Bodies and Practices of Carnie Wilson and Anna Nicole Smith" (paper, International Communication Association Conference, New York, 2005); Le'a Kent, "Fighting Abjection: Representing Fat Women," in *Bodies Out of Bounds: Fatness and Transgression*, ed. Jana Evans Braziel and Kathleen LeBesco (Berkeley: University of California Press, 2001), 130–145.

17. Gareth Palmer, "Legitimate Targets: Reality Television and Large People," in *Reality Gendervision: Sexuality and Gender on Transatlantic Reality Television*, ed. Brenda Weber (Durham, N.C.: Duke University Press, 2014), 302.

18. June Deery, "Interior Design: Commodifying Self and Place in *Extreme Makeover, Extreme Makeover: Home Edition*, and *The Swan*," in Heller, *Great American Makeover*, 168.

19. Ibid.

20. Andrew Dugan, "Fast Food Still Major Part of U.S. Diet," Gallup, August 6, 2013, www .gallup.com/poll/163868/fast-food-major-part-diet.aspx.

21. Alan Warde and Lydia Martens, *Eating Out: Social Differentiation, Consumption, and Pleasure* (Cambridge: Cambridge University Press, 2000).

22. Cathy Banwell, Dorothy Broom, Anna Davis, and Jane Dixon, *Weight of Modernity: An Intergenerational Study of the Rise of Obesity* (New York: Springer, 2012).

23. These television tales of sacrificial motherhood resemble Susan Douglas's concept of "new momism," which is the idealization of an "intensive motherhood" that makes it difficult

for women to focus on their own needs and desires. See Douglas, *The Mommy Myth* (New York: Free Press, 2005).

24. Brenda Weber, *Makeover TV: Selfhood, Citizenship, and Celebrity* (Durham, N.C.: Duke University Press, 2009), 83–92.

25. Palmer, "Legitimate Targets," 305.

26. Weber, *Makeover TV*, 87.

27. Weber, *Makeover TV*; Palmer, "Legitimate Targets"; and Martin Roberts, "The Fashion Police and Governing the Self in *What Not To Wear*," in *Interrogating Post-Feminism*, ed. Yvonne Tasker and Diane Negra (Durham, N.C.: Duke University Press, 2007), 227–248.

28. "The Biggest Loser May Be the Viewer," *Globe and Mail*, October 19, 2007.

29. Weber, *Makeover TV*, 84.

30. Deborah Lupton, *Fat* (New York: Routledge, 2013); Kathleen LeBesco, "Fat Panic and the New Morality," in *Against Health: How Health Became the New Morality*, ed. Jonathan M. Metzl and Anna Kirkland (New York: New York University Press, 2010), 72–82; Abigail Saguy, *What's Wrong with Fat?* (Oxford: Oxford University Press, 2013).

31. Palmer, "Legitimate Targets," 313.

32. Weber, *Makeover TV*, 73.

33. Fell, "'It's a Miracle No One Has Died Yet.'"

34. Weber, *Makeover TV*, 104.

35. Ibid., 111–112.

36. Ibid., 113.

37. Former participants on *Extreme Weight Loss* dispute that Powell actually ever moves in with them.

38. Palmer, "Legitimate Targets," 313.

39. Ibid., 313.

40. Maureen Callahan, "'We're All Fat Again': More 'Biggest Loser' Contestants Reveal Secrets," *New York Post*, January 25, 2015, http://nypost.com/2015/01/25/were-all-fat-again-more-biggest-loser-contestants-reveal-secrets/.

41. Wyatt, "On 'The Biggest Loser.'"

42. Lindsey Bever, "'I Feel Embarrassed': A 'Biggest Loser' Winner Confesses Her Weight-Gain Shame," *Washington Post*, April 29, 2016.

43. Lisa Respers France, "'Biggest Loser' Winner Talks Regaining the Weight," *CNN*, April 27, 2016.

44. Ibid.

45. Gina Kolata, "After 'The Biggest Loser,' Their Bodies Fought to Regain Weight," *New York Times*, May 2, 2016, www.nytimes.com/2016/05/02/health/biggest-loser-weight-loss.html?smid=fb-nytimes&smtyp=cur&_r=2.

46. Weber, *Makeover TV*, 99.

47. Roberts, "Fashion Police," 245.

48. Eliana Dockterman, "'Biggest Loser' Winner Rachel Frederickson Admits She May Have Gone Too Far," *Time*, February 12, 2014, http://time.com/6739/biggest-loser-winner-rachel-frederickson-admits-she-may-have-gone-too-far/.

49. Jacque Wilson and Emily Hayes, "'Biggest Loser' Winner: Too Thin?" *CNN*, February 6, 2014, www.cnn.com/2014/02/05/health/biggest-weight-loss/; Kasey Edwards, "Shamed for Being Fat, Then for Being Thin," *Stuff*, July 2, 2014, www.stuff.co.nz/life-style/wellbeing/9696183/Shamed-for-being-fat-then-for-being-thin; "'Biggest Loser' Winner Rachel Frederickson

Says She May Have Gone Too Far," *Huffington Post*, February 12, 2014, www.huffingtonpost .com/2014/02/12/biggest-loser-too-far_n_4775103.html.

50. Fell, "'It's a Miracle No One Has Died Yet.'"

51. Tanya Berry et al., "Effects of Biggest Loser Exercise Depictions on Exercise-Related Attitudes," *American Journal of Behavioral Health* 37, no. 1 (2013): 96–103.

52. Tanya Berry comments on her study, "Effects of Biggest Loser Exercise Depictions on Exercise-Related Attitudes," in Yoni Freedhoff, "When Science Met the Biggest Loser," *U.S. News & World Report*, January 23, 2013, http://health.usnews.com/health-news/blogs/eat -run/2013/01/23/when-science-met-the-biggest-loser.

CHAPTER 6 — SPECTACLE, SYMPATHY, AND THE MEDICALIZED DISEASE OF "OBESITY"

1. Holly Baxter, "If You Think the Autopsy of a Fat Woman on TV Will Solve the Obesity Epidemic, You're Wrong," *Independent*, September 14, 2016, www.independent.co.uk/voices /obesity-the-post-mortem-autopsy-of-fat-woman-obese-solve-epidemic-here-is-why-youre -wrong-a7307251.html.

2. Ibid.; Helen Archer, "So Much Fat!—The Cruel Autopsy of a 17-Stone Woman on the BBC," *Guardian*, September 13, 2016, www.theguardian.com/tv-and-radio/2016/sep/13 /obesity-the-post-mortem-so-much-fat-the-cruel-autopsy-of-a-17–stone-woman-bbc.

3. Beverley Skeggs and Helen Wood, *Reacting to Reality Television: Performance, Audience, and Value* (New York: Routledge, 2012), 104; Simon Brown and Stacy Abbott, "The Art of Sp(l)atter: Body Horror in *Dexter*," in *Dexter: Investigating Cutting Edge Television*, ed. Simon Brown and Stacy Abbott (London: I.B. Taurus, 2010), 208.

4. Jason Jacobs, *Body Trauma TV: The New Hospital Dramas* (London: BFI, 2003), 68.

5. Helen Wheatley, *Spectacular Television: Exploring Televisual Pleasure* (London: I.B. Taurus, 2016), 13.

6. "*My 600-lb Life* Season 5" (Discovery Communications press release, 2017), https://press .discovery.com/us/tlc/programs/my-600–lb-life-season-5/.

7. Susan Murray, "'I Think We Need a New Name for It': The Meeting of Documentary and Reality TV," in *Reality TV: Remaking Television Culture*, 2nd ed., ed. Susan Murray and Laurie Ouellette (New York: New York University Press, 2009), 40–55.

8. Jason Mittell, "A Cultural Approach to Television Genre Theory," *Cinema Journal* 40, no. 3 (2001): 3–24.

9. Lawrence Grossberg, *We Gotta Get Out of This Place: Popular Conservatism and Postmodern Culture* (London: Routledge, 1992), 84.

10. Wheatley, *Spectacular Television*, 156; Katherine Sender and Margaret Sullivan, "Epidemics of Will, Failures of Self-Esteem: Responding to Fat Bodies in *The Biggest Loser* and *What Not to Wear*," *Continuum* 22, no. 4 (2008): 573–584.

11. Robert Pollack Seid, *Never Too Thin* (New York: Prentice Hall, 1989), 22.

12. Cited in Thomas Osborne, "On Anti-medicine and Clinical Reason," in *Reassessing Foucault: Power, Medicine, and the Body*, ed. Colin Jones and Roy Porter (New York: Routledge, 1998), 31.

13. David Armstrong, "Bodies of Knowledge/Knowledge of Bodies," in Jones and Porter, *Reassessing Foucault*, 11–12.

14. Nikolas Rose, "Medicine, History, and the Present," in Jones and Porter, *Reassessing Foucault*, 64.

15. Ibid., 51.

16. Julie Elman, "After School Special Education: Rehabilitative Television, Teen Citizenship, and Compulsory Able-Bodiedness," *Television and New Media* 11, no. 4 (2010): 261.

17. George Gerbner, Larry Gross, Michael Morgan, and Nancy Signorielli, "Health and Medicine on Television," *New England Journal of Medicine* 305 (1981): 903.

18. Joseph Turow, *Playing Doctor: Television, Storytelling, and Medical Power* (Ann Arbor: University of Michigan Press, 1989), 106.

19. Gregory Makoul and Limor Peer, "Dissecting the Doctor Shows: A Content Analysis of *ER* and *Chicago Hope*," in *Cultural Sutures: Medicine and Media*, ed. Lester D. Friedman (Durham, N.C.: Duke University Press, 2004), 244.

20. Nikola Rose, "Medicine, History, and the Present," 56, 69.

21. Turow, *Playing Doctor*, 29.

22. Marc R. Cohen and Audrey Shafer, "Images and Healers: A Visual History of Scientific Medicine," in Friedman, *Cultural Sutures*, 201.

23. John Dempsey, "Health Net Builds Fla. Complex," *Daily Variety*, August 8, 1995.

24. Lester D. Friedman, "Introduction: Through the Looking Glass: Medical Culture and the Media," in Friedman, *Cultural Sutures*, 2.

25. Dorothy Nelkin, *Selling Science: How the Press Covers Science and Technology* (London: Freeman, 1987).

26. Peter Conrad, "The Shifting Engines of Medicalization," *Journal of Health and Social Behavior* 46 (2005): 3–14.

27. Christina Korowynk, Michael R. Kolber, James McCormack, Vanessa Lam, Kate Overbo, Candra Cotton, Caitlin Finley, Ricky D. Turgeon, Scott Garrison, Adrienne J. Lindblad, Hoan Linh Banh, Denise Campbell-Schere, Ben Vandermeer, and G. Michael Allan, "Televised Medical Talk Shows—What They Recommend and the Evidence to Support Their Recommendations: A Prospective Observational Study," *BMJ* 349 (2014): 1–9.

28. Jen Christensen and Jacque Wilson, "Congressional Hearing Investigates Dr. Oz 'Miracle' Weight Loss Claims," *CNN*, June 19, 2014, www.cnn.com/2014/06/17/health/senate-grills-dr-oz/.

29. "Marketer Who Promoted a Green Coffee Bean Weight-Loss Supplement Agrees to Settle FTC Charges" (Federal Trade Commission press release, January 26, 2015), www.ftc.gov/news-events/press-releases/2015/01/marketer-who-promoted-green-coffee-bean-weight-loss-supplement.

30. Mark Andrejevic, *Infoglut: How Too Much Information Is Changing the Way We Think and Know* (New York: Routledge, 2013).

31. Kristen Houghton, "A Snake Oil Salesman Alive and Well in Dr. Oz," *Huffington Post*, June 30, 2014, www.huffingtonpost.com/kristen-houghton/snakeoil-salesman-alive-a_b_5537666.html.

32. Kiera Butler, "When Medical Apps Do More Harm Than Good," *Mother Jones*, January 5, 2015, www.motherjones.com/environment/2015/01/medical-apps-not-helping.

33. Deborah Lupton, "Foucault and the Medicalization Critique," in *Foucault, Health, and Medicine*, ed. Alan Peterson and Robin Bunton (London: Routledge, 1997), 102.

34. Michel Foucault, "'The Confession of the Flesh' 1977 Interview," in *Power/Knowledge: Selected Interviews and Other Writings by Michel Foucault*, ed. Colin Gordon (New York: Pantheon Books, 1980), 56.

35. Helen Wheatley, *Spectacular Television*, 174.

36. Myra Mendible, "High Theory/Low Culture: Postmodernism and the Politics of the Carnival," *Journal of American Culture* 22, no. 2 (1999): 74.

37. Francis Bonner, *Ordinary Television: Analyzing Popular TV* (London: Sage, 2003), 114; José Van Dijck, "The Endoscopic Gaze," *International Journal of Cultural Studies* 4, no. 2 (2001): 219–237.

38. Michel Foucault, *Discipline and Punish: The Birth of Prison* (New York: Vintage, 1979), 58.

39. Tony Bennett, "The Exhibitionary Complex," *New Formations* 4 (1998): 85.

40. Foucault, *Discipline and Punish*, 59 and 63.

41. Michael Silk, Jessica Francombe, and F. Bachelor, "*The Biggest Loser*: The Discursive Constitution of Fatness," *Interactions: Studies in Communication and Culture* 1, no. 3 (2009): 369–389; Cressida Heyes, *Self-Transformations: Foucault, Ethics, and Normalized Bodies* (Oxford: Oxford University Press, 2007); Martin Roberts, "The Fashion Police and Governing the Self in *What Not To Wear*," in *Interrogating Post-Feminism*, ed. Yvonne Tasker and Diane Negra (Durham, N.C.: Duke University Press, 2007), 227–248; Gareth Palmer, "Video Vigilantes and the Work of Shame," *Jump Cut* 48 (2006), www.ejumpcut.org/archive/jc48.2006/shameTV/.

42. José van Dijck, "Medical Documentary: Conjoined Twins as a Mediated Spectacle," *Media, Culture & Society* 24 (2002): 537–556; Sarah Kember, "Medicine's New Vision?," in *The Photographic Image in Digital Culture*, ed. M. Lister (London: Routledge), 95–114.

43. Van Dijck, "Endoscopic Gaze," 226.

44. David Lyon, *Theorizing Surveillance: The Panopticon and Beyond* (Cullompton: Willan, 2006), 8.

45. Brenda Weber, *Makeover TV: Selfhood, Citizenship, and Celebrity* (Durham, N.C.: Duke University Press, 2009), 97.

46. Gareth Palmer, "Legitimate Targets: Reality Television and Large People," in *Reality Gendervision: Sexuality and Gender on Transatlantic Reality Television*, ed. Brenda Weber (Durham, N.C.: Duke University Press, 2014), 303.

47. Hannah Frith, Jayne Raisborough, and Orly Klein, "Shame and Pride in *How to Look Good Naked*: The Affective Dynamics of (Mis)Recognition," *Feminist Media Studies* 14, no. 2 (2012): 165–177; Jennifer Fremline, "The Weigh-In as a National Money Shot," *Flow* 7, no. 13 (2008), www.flowjournal.org/2008/05/extreme-biggest-celebrity-fit-loser-makeover-club-the-weigh-in-as-national-money-shot/.

48. Jeff Jervis, *Sympathetic Sentiments: Affect, Emotion, and Spectacle in the Modern World* (London: Bloomsbury, 2015), 101.

49. Ibid., 7.

50. Tiara Sukhan, "Bootcamps, Brides, and BMI: Biopedagogical Narratives of Health and Belonging on Canadian Size-Transformation Television," *Television & New Media* 14, no. 3 (2012): 198.

51. Palmer, "Legitimate Targets," 302.

52. Weber, *Makeover TV*, 97.

53. Palmer, "Video Vigilantes"; Weber, *Makeover TV*, 98.

54. Alison Bonaguro, "This Is One of the Biggest Weight-Loss Lessons You Can Learn from 'My 600-Pound Life,'" *Women's Health*, August 8, 2017, www.womenshealthmag.com/weight-loss/friends-and-family-sabotage-weight-loss-goals.

55. Douglas Kellner, "Media Culture and the Triumph of Spectacle," in *The Spectacle of the Real: From Hollywood to Reality TV and Beyond*, ed. Geoff King (Bristol: Intellect, 2005), 29.

56. Patricia Hughes-Fuller, "Wild Bodies and True Lies: Carnival, Spectacle, and the Curious Case of *Trailer Park Boy*," *Canadian Journal of Communication* 34 (2009): 99.

57. Deborah Lupton, *Fat* (New York: Routledge, 2013), 25.

58. Weber, *Makeover TV*, 111–113.

59. Palmer, "Legitimate Targets," 313.

60. Ralph DiLeone, Jane R. Taylor, and Marina R. Picciotto, "The Drive to Eat: Comparisons and Distinctions between Mechanisms of Food Reward and Drug Addiction," *Nature Neuroscience* 15 (2012): 1330–1335.

61. Maria Vultaggio, "Dr. Nowzaradan's Diet Plan for 'My 600 Pound Life' Patients: How TLC Reality Stars Lose Weight after Gastric Bypass," *International Business Times*, January 3, 2017, www.ibtimes.com/dr-nowzaradans-diet-plan-my-600-lb-life-patients-how-tlc-reality-stars-lose-weight-2468821.

62. A. P. Courcoulas, N. J. Christian, S. H. Belle, et al., "Weight Change and Health Outcomes at 3 Years after Bariatric Surgery among Individuals with Severe Obesity," *Journal of the American Medical Association* 310, no. 22 (2013): 2416–2425.

63. Alisha M. Wade, "Fatal Malnutrition 6 Years after Gastric Bypass Surgery," *Journal of the American Medical Association* 170, no. 11 (2010): 993–995.

64. Patrick D. Hahn, "Cutting Edge: Bariatric Surgery May Do More Harm Than Good," *Baltimore Sun*, April 12, 2017, www.baltimoresun.com/news/opinion/oped/bs-ed-bariatric-surgery-20170412-story.html.

65. Brittany King, "*My 600-LB. Life* Stars Open Up about the Hardest Part of Losing Weight: 'The Cravings Are Still There,'" *People*, May 25, 2017, http://people.com/bodies/my-600-lb-life-stars-open-up-hardest-part-losing-weight-cravings/.

66. Gina Kolata, "After Weight-Loss Surgery, a Year of Joys and Disappointments," *New York Times*, December 27, 2016, www.nytimes.com/2016/12/27/health/bariatric-surgery.html?rref=collection%2Fseriescollection%2FThe%20Science%20of%20Fat&_r=1.

67. Weber, *Makeover TV*, 82.

68. Bonner, *Ordinary Television*, 112–113.

69. Kathleen LeBesco, "Fat Panic and the New Morality," in *Against Health: How Health Became the New Morality*, ed. Jonathan M. Metzl and Anna Kirkland (New York: New York University Press, 2010), 78.

CHAPTER 7 — CELEBRATING LARGE BODIES ON THE SMALL SCREEN

1. Kimberly Dark, "Why You Should Love and Hate the Louis CK 'Fat Girl Rant'—And What to Do about It," *Huffington Post*, May 22, 2014, www.huffingtonpost.com/kimberly-dark/louis-ck-fat-girl-rant-episode_b_5361261.html.

2. Madeleine Davies, "Louis C.K.'s Rant on Fat Girls Is Absolutely Magnificent," *Jezebel*, May 13, 2014, http://jezebel.com/louis-c-k-s-rant-on-fat-girls-is-absolutely-magnificent-1575653738.

3. Willa Paskin, "Louie Has No Idea What It's Like to Be a 'Fat Girl.' Neither Does Louis CK," *Slate*, May 12, 2014, www.slate.com/blogs/xx_factor/2014/05/12/louie_so_did_the_fat_lady_louis_ck_writes_a_fat_girl_to_apologize_for_men.html.

4. Alex Strachan, "Dispelling the Myth TV Is Only about the Skinny; Plus-Sized Partners Live Out Real-Life Problems on the Funny Mike and Molly," *Edmonton Journal*, March 20, 2011.

5. Cathy Young, "Pro-Fat an Unhealthy Status Quo," *Boston Globe*, December 30, 2013, www.bostonglobe.com/opinion/2013/12/30/fat-acceptance-hazardous-health/10jfoW46R2elWpHLarA19M/story.html.

6. Arlene Vigoda, "In Practice, Manheim Wakes Up World with Weighty Matters," *USA Today*, May 11, 2011.

7. Timothy Havens, "Towards a Structuration Theory of Media Intermediaries," in *Making Media Work: Cultures of Management in the Entertainment Industry*, ed. Derek Johnson, Derek Kompare, and Avi Santo (New York: New York University Press, 2014), 39.

8. Ibid., 51; Timothy Havens, *Black Television Travels: African American Media around the Globe* (New York: New York University Press, 2014).

9. Havens, "Towards a Structuration Theory," 60.

10. Julie D'Acci, *Defining Women: Television and the Case of Cagney and Lacey* (Chapel Hill: University of North Carolina Press, 1994); Christine Acham, *Revolution Televised: Prime Time and the Struggle for Black Power* (Minneapolis: University of Minnesota Press, 2005).

11. Samantha Kwan and Jennifer Graves, *Framing Fat: Competing Constructions in Contemporary Culture* (New Brunswick, N.J.: Rutgers University Press, 2013), 39.

12. Allison Hope Weiner, "Fall TV Schedule Gorges on Weight-Loss Shows," *Hollywood Reporter*, September 16, 2010.

13. Ibid.

14. Michael Schneider, "Reality TV Continues Fascination with Fat," *Variety*, July 25, 2009, http://variety.com/2009/tv/news/reality-tv-continues-fascination-with-fat-1118006475/.

15. Ibid.

16. "'Huge' Marks Advance for Fat Acceptance in Hollywood," *Times of Oman*, June 30, 2010.

17. Schneider, "Reality TV Continues Fascination with Fat."

18. Rob Owens, "More to Love on TV; Shows Focusing on Obese People after Success of 'The Biggest Loser," *Pittsburgh Post-Gazette*, July 12, 2009.

19. Ginia Bellafante, "A Sitcom with More Than Empty Calories," *New York Times*, September 20, 2010.

20. Megan Angelo, "The Mindy Project's Mindy Lahiri Is Our Self-Image Idol," *Glamour*, October 7, 2014, www.glamour.com/entertainment/blogs/obsessed/2014/10/why-the-mindy-projects-mindy-l.

21. Sheila Moeschen, "What 'The Mindy Project' Gets Right about Body Image," *Huffington Post*, April 25, 2013, www.huffingtonpost.com/sheila-moeschen/what-the-mindy-project-gets-right-about-body-image_b_3155072.html.

22. Laura S. Brown, "Fat-Oppressive Attitudes and the Feminist Therapist: Directions for Change," in *Fat Oppression and Psychotherapy: A Feminist Perspective*, ed. Laura S. Brown and Esther D. Rothblum (New York: Hawthorne Press, 1989), 19–30.

23. Matthew Gilbert, "The Naked Truth about Lena Dunham's Fresh Body of Work," *Boston Globe*, March 22, 2014, www.bostonglobe.com/arts/television/2014/03/22/lena-dunham-idea-lena-dunham/9nPonyTBNg0fTMpfYbAbWM/story.html; Fariha Rosen, "What's My Body Got to Do with It? Body and Beauty Standards and What Lena Dunham Is Doing for It All," *Huffington Post*, February 22, 2013, www.huffingtonpost.com/fariha-roisin/lena-dunham-body-image_b_2721796.html; Moeschen, "What 'The Mindy Project' Gets Right about Body Image"; Emily Nussbaum, "It's Different for 'Girls,'" *New York Magazine*, March, 25, 2012, http://nymag.com/arts/tv/features/girls-lena-dunham-2012-4/index1.html.

24. Stephanie Weber, "Joan Rivers Slams Lena Dunham's Body Positive Message: 'Stay Fat,' 'Get Diabetes,'" *US Weekly*, March 26, 2014, www.usmagazine.com/celebrity-news/news/joan-rivers-slams-lena-dunhams-body-positive-message-stay-fat-get-diabetes-2014263.

25. Julia Sonenshein, "Lena Dunham's Type of Body Acceptance Isn't Doing Us Any Favors," *Gloss*, May 13, 2014, www.thegloss.com/2014/05/13/beauty/lena-dunham-body-acceptance-bad/#ixzz3OSXrsvui.

26. Elissa Strauss, "Why Mindy Kaling—Not Lena Dunham—Is the Body Positive Icon of the Moment," *Week*, April 22, 2014, http://theweek.com/articles/447722/mindy-kaling—lena-dunham—body-positive-icon-moment.

27. Andrew Hampp, "Latest Crop of Plus-Size TV Aims to Win by Not Focusing on Losing," *Advertising Age*, July 12, 2010, http://adage.com/article/media/tv-huge-mike-molly-lighter-approach-weight/144866/.

28. David Hinckley, "They Don't Fit the Profile: TV Takes a More Rounded View of the Overweight," *New York Daily News*, October 17, 2010.

29. Emily Yah, "Beauty & the Burden: 'Diva's' Got Hefty Issues," *Washington Post*, July 25, 2009.

30. Hampp, "Latest Crop of Plus-Size TV."

31. Yah, "Beauty & the Burden."

32. Fat bodies are often considered a "before" state rather than a "future" state, positioning fat bodies as nonhuman or as "encasing a human." See Le'a Kent, "Fighting Abjection: Representing Fat Women," in *Bodies Out of Bounds: Fatness and Transgression*, ed. Jana Evans Braziel and Kathleen LeBesco (Berkeley: University of California Press, 2001), 130–145.

33. Cristina Kinon, "'Drop Dead Diva' Actress Brooke Elliott Says Plus Size Isn't a Minus," *New York Daily News*, June 17, 2009, www.nydailynews.com/entertainment/tv-movies/drop-dead-diva-actress-brooke-elliott-size-isn-article-1.375354.

34. Tara Parker-Pope, "Getting Real about Weight: TV Drama Recasts Issue; Personal Health," *International Herald Tribune*, September 24, 2009.

35. Gina Belafonte, "Can Girls Be Overweight and Not Overwrought?," *New York Times*, June 27, 2010, https://www.nytimes.com/2010/06/28/arts/television/28huge.html.

36. Jessica Bennett, "ABC Family's New Fat Camp Drama, 'Huge,'" *Newsweek*, June 27, 2010, www.newsweek.com/tv-review-abc-familys-new-fat-camp-drama-huge-73551.

37. Bill Keveney, "ABC Family's 'Huge' Tackles Issues of Teen Obesity," *USA Today*, June 28, 2010, http://usatoday30.usatoday.com/life/television/news/2010-06-28-huge28_ST_N.htm.

38. Ibid.

39. Coeli Carr, "TV's New Sitcom 'Mike & Molly': Are Its Fat Jokes Funny or Offensive?" *ABC News*, September 28, 2010, http://abcnews.go.com/Entertainment/mike-molly-fat-jokes-funny-offensive/story?id=11692329#.Ucx3Hvb8kt; Joel Keller, "The Only Thing Offensive about Mike and Molly Is the Fat Jokes," *Huffpost TV*, October 27, 2010, www.aoltv.com/2010/10/27/the-only-thing-offensive-about-mike-and-molly-is-the-fat-jokes/; Kevin Fallon, "'Mike and Molly' vs. 'Outsource': Which New Series Is More Offensive?," *Atlantic*, September 25, 2010, www.theatlantic.com/entertainment/archive/2010/09/mike-molly-vs-outsourced-which-new-series-is-more-offensive/63547/.

40. Julie Miller, "The Mike and Molly Fat Joke Tracker: You Were Eating Corn on the Cob Before You Had Teeth," *Movieline*, October 5, 2010, http://movieline.com/2010/10/05/the-mike-molly-fat-joke-tracker-you-were-eating-corn-on-the-cob-before-you-had-teeth/.

41. Dina Giovanelli and Stephen Osterag, "Controlling the Body: Media Representations, Body Size, and Self-Discipline,'" in *The Fat Studies Reader*, ed. Esther Rothblum and Sondra Solovay (New York: New York University, 2009), 289–299.

42. Bellafante, "A Sitcom with More Than Empty Calories."

43. David Hickley, "'Mike & Molly' Avoids Heavy-Handed Fat Jokes in Favor of Big-Hearted Laughs," *New York Daily News*, September 20, 2010, http://www.nydailynews.com/entertainment/tv-movies/mike-molly-avoids-heavy-handed-fat-jokes-favor-big-hearted-laughs-article-1.441798.

44. Alex Strachan, "Dispelling the Myth TV Is Only about the Skinny; Plus-Sized Partners Live Out Real-Life Problems on the Funny Mike and Molly," *Edmonton Journal*, March 20, 2011.

45. Ann Oldenburg, "Star of 'Mike & Molly' Says Success Is Worth the Weight; To Comic Billy Gardell, Humor Comes from Caring," *USA Today*, October 3, 2011.

46. Kwan and Graves, *Framing Fat*, 50–53.

47. Interview with Bruce David Klein, 2013.

48. Interview with Tiffany Banks, 2013.

49. Sydney Bucksbaum, "Nicole Byer Won't Apologize for Her Comedy (But She'll Always Read the Comments," *Hollywood Reporter*, August 29, 2016, www.hollywoodreporter .com/live-feed/nicole-byer-loosely-exactly-nicole-921599.

50. Thomas Streeter, *Selling the Air: A Critique of the Policy of Commercial Broadcasting in the United States* (Chicago: University of Chicago Press, 1996), 115–117.

CONCLUSION

1. Edward Wyatt, "On 'The Biggest Loser,' Health Can Take a Back Seat," *New York Times*, November 24, 2009, www.nytimes.com/2009/11/25/business/media/25loser.html?mtrref =undefined.

2. Similar eating issues are addressed with Alyssa on *Extreme Weight Loss* and Shay on *Thintervention*.

3. Maureen Callahan, "'We're All Fat Again': More 'Biggest Loser' Contestants Reveal Secrets," *New York Post*, January 25, 2015, http://nypost.com/2015/01/25/were-all-fat-again -more-biggest-loser-contestants-reveal-secrets/.

4. Ibid.

5. Alex Stedman, "'Biggest Loser' Under Inquiry by Los Angeles Sherriff's Department for Drug Allegations," *Variety*, May 31, 2016, http://variety.com/2016/tv/news/biggest -loser-drug-investigation-sheriffs-department-1201786005/.

6. Jason Brow, "'The Biggest Loser' Scandal: Former Contestant Claims Trainer Forced Her to Take Drugs," *Hollywood Life*, May 23, 2016, http://hollywoodlife.com/2016/05/23 /biggest-loser-drug-scandal-joelle-gwynn-bob-harper/.

7. Wyatt, "On 'The Biggest Loser."

8. "'Biggest Loser' Shocker: Jillian Michaels Did a Bad, Bad Thing," *Yahoo! TV*, November 13, 2013, www.yahoo.com/tv/bp/biggest-loser—shocker—jillian-michaels-did-a-bad— bad-thing-093656195.html?nf=1.

9. Yoni Freedhoff, "The Real Biggest Losers? The Show's Audience," *Huffington Post*, March 16, 2013, www.huffingtonpost.ca/yoni-freedhoff/biggest-loser-kids-_b_2473934.html.

10. American Council on Exercise, "American Council on Exercise Tackles the Reality of Reality TV Weight Loss," *Physician Business Week*, April 2, 2013, 238.

11. William Anderson, "The Biggest Loser: Rated 'X,'" *McClathy- Tribune Business News*, May 10, 2010.

12. Erin Fothergill et al., "Persistent Metabolic Adaptation 6 Years after 'The Biggest Loser' Competition," *Obesity: A Research Journal* 24, no. 8 (2016): 1612–1619.

13. Gina Kolata, "After 'The Biggest Loser,' Their Bodies Fought to Regain Weight," *New York Times*, May 2, 2016, www.nytimes.com/2016/05/02/health/biggest-loser-weight-loss .html?smid=fb-nytimes&smtyp=cur&_r=2.

14. Wyatt, "On 'The Biggest Loser.'"

15. "JD Roth Chats New Book and Weight Loss Show," *Z Living*, May 18, 2016, www.zliving .com/fitness/weight-loss/jd-roth.

16. Ibid.

17. Erin Brodwin, "A New Show Features 'Biggest Loser' Winners Who Regained Weight— And Reveals a Deeper Truth about Weight Loss," *Business Insider*, June 11, 2017, www .businessinsider.com/new-show-biggest-loser-winners-regained-weight-big-fat-truth-2017-6.

18. Brandon Ambrosino, "The Tyranny of Buffness," *Atlantic*, August 16, 2013, www
.theatlantic.com/sexes/archive/2013/08/the-tyranny-of-buffness/278698/.

19. Jonathan M. Metzl, "Introduction: Why 'Against Health'?," in *Against Health: How
Health Became the New Morality*, ed. Jonathan M. Metzl and Anna Kirkland (New York: New
York University Press, 2010), 3–4.

Index

Photos, figures, and tables are indicated by italicized page number.

About the Author

Melissa Zimdars is an assistant professor of communication and media at Merrimack College. She earned her Ph.D. from the University of Iowa in communication studies, and her M.A. and B.A. from the University of Wisconsin–Milwaukee.